CARB CYCLING COOK BOOK FOR SENIORS

Complete Guide For Weight Loss And Delicious Recipes

For Optimal Health

MAI STEPHEN

Copyright © 2023

All Rights Are Reserved

The content in this book may not be reproduced, duplicated, or transferred without the express written permission of the author or publisher. Under no circumstances will the publisher or author be held liable or legally responsible for any losses, expenditures, or damages incurred directly or indirectly as a consequence of the information included in this book.

Legal Remarks

Copyright protection applies to this publication. It is only intended for personal use. No piece of this work may be modified, distributed, sold, quoted, or paraphrased without the author's or publisher's consent.

Disclaimer Statement

Please keep in mind that the contents of this booklet are meant for educational and recreational purposes. Every effort has been made to offer accurate, up-to-date, reliable, and thorough information. There are, however, no stated or implied assurances of any kind. Readers understand that the author is providing competent counsel. The content in this book originates from several sources. Please seek the opinion of a competent professional before using any of the tactics outlined in this book. By reading this book, the reader agrees that the author will not be held accountable for any direct or indirect damages resulting from the use of the information contained therein, including, but not limited to, errors, omissions, or inaccuracies

Contents

INTRODUCTION

In the pursuit of health and fitness, individuals are constantly bombarded with a multitude of dietary strategies, each promising remarkable result. Among these approaches, carb cycling has emerged as a popular and effective method for achieving various health and fitness goals. While initially embraced by athletes and fitness enthusiasts, its potential benefits for seniors have increasingly come to light in recent years. Carb cycling revolves around the manipulation of carbohydrate intake, alternating between high and low-carb days over a specified period. This dietary strategy aims to optimize energy levels, enhance fat loss, and support muscle growth by strategically adjusting carbohydrate consumption.

For seniors, carb cycling offers a unique opportunity to tailor their dietary approach to meet the specific challenges and requirements of aging. As individuals grow older, their nutritional needs and metabolic processes undergo significant changes, necessitating a more nuanced approach to diet and nutrition. Traditional dietary recommendations may not adequately address the unique needs of seniors, leaving many searchings for alternative strategies to support their health and fitness goals. In this chapter, we will explore the fundamentals of carb cycling for seniors, shedding light on its potential benefits and practical applications in the context of aging.

Understanding Carb Cycling

Carb cycling is a dietary approach that involves alternating between periods of high and low carbohydrate intake. The premise behind carb cycling is to strategically manipulate carb intake to maximize energy levels, optimize performance, and promote fat loss while minimizing negative side effects associated with sustained low-carb diets.

For seniors, understanding the principles of carb cycling is crucial for maintaining overall health and well-being. As we age, our metabolism tends to slow down, and we may become more susceptible to insulin resistance and other metabolic issues. Carb cycling offers a flexible and sustainable way to manage blood sugar levels, improve insulin sensitivity, and support healthy aging.

The concept of carb cycling revolves around the idea of timing carbohydrate intake based on activity levels and metabolic needs. On high activity days, such as during exercise or physical exertion, seniors may benefit from consuming a higher proportion of carbohydrates to fuel their activities and replenish glycogen stores. Conversely, on rest days or days with lower activity levels, reducing carbohydrate intake can help prevent excess calorie consumption and promote fat burning.

One of the key aspects of carb cycling is its individualized nature. Seniors may need to experiment with different carb cycling protocols to find what works best for their bodies and goals. Factors such as age, activity level, metabolic rate, and overall health should be taken into consideration when designing a carb cycling plan.

It's also essential to note that carb cycling is not a one-size-fits-all approach. Some seniors may thrive on a more aggressive carb cycling regimen, while others may prefer a more moderate approach. Consulting with a healthcare professional or registered dietitian can help seniors determine the most appropriate carb cycling strategy for their needs.

Benefits of Carb Cycling for Seniors

Carb cycling offers a myriad of potential benefits for seniors, ranging from improved metabolic health to enhanced physical performance and mental clarity. By strategically manipulating carbohydrate intake, seniors can unlock a host of advantages that contribute to overall well-being and quality of life.

One of the primary benefits of carb cycling for seniors is its ability to regulate blood sugar levels and improve insulin sensitivity. As we age, our bodies may become less efficient at processing carbohydrates, leading to fluctuations in blood sugar and increased risk of insulin resistance and type 2 diabetes. By cycling carbohydrates, seniors can help stabilize blood sugar levels, reduce insulin spikes, and promote better metabolic health.

Furthermore, carb cycling can support weight management and body composition goals in seniors. By alternating between high and low carbohydrate days, seniors can create a calorie deficit while preserving lean muscle mass. This can be especially beneficial for seniors looking to lose excess body fat or maintain a healthy weight as they age.

In addition to its metabolic benefits, carb cycling can also enhance physical performance and recovery in seniors. Consuming adequate carbohydrates on high activity days provides the energy necessary to fuel workouts and support muscle repair and recovery. On the other hand, reducing carbohydrate intake on rest days can help seniors avoid feelings of sluggishness and fatigue often associated with carb-heavy meals.

Another notable benefit of carb cycling for seniors is its potential impact on cognitive function and brain health. Research suggests that carbohydrates play a vital role in brain function, and inadequate carb intake can impair cognitive performance and memory. By incorporating strategic carb cycling into their diet, seniors can ensure they're providing their brains with the fuel needed to stay sharp and focused.

Moreover, carb cycling offers seniors a flexible and sustainable approach to nutrition that can be easily tailored to individual preferences and lifestyle factors. Unlike strict low-carb diets, which can be challenging to maintain long-term, carb cycling allows seniors to enjoy a variety of foods while still achieving their health and fitness goals.

How Carb Cycling Supports Senior Health and Fitness

Carb cycling holds immense promise for seniors seeking to optimize their health and fitness in later life. By strategically manipulating carbohydrate intake, seniors can unlock a myriad smetabolic flexibility to promoting weight management, carb cycling offers a multifaceted approach to senior health and fitness that addresses the unique challenges of aging.

One of the key ways in which carb cycling supports senior health and fitness is through its impact on metabolism. As individuals age, metabolic rate tends to decline, making it increasingly challenging to maintain a healthy weight and body composition. By cycling between periods of high and low-carbohydrate intake, seniors can effectively modulate their metabolic rate, promoting fat loss while preserving lean muscle mass. This not only aids in weight management but also enhances metabolic health, reducing the risk of obesity-related diseases such as type 2 diabetes and cardiovascular disease.

Furthermore, carb cycling can improve insulin sensitivity and glycsemic control, which are crucial factors in maintaining overall health and well-being in seniors. By reducing carbohydrate intake on low-carb days, seniors can minimize spikes in blood sugar levels, thereby reducing the risk of insulin resistance and related complications. This is particularly relevant for seniors at risk of or managing type 2 diabetes, as carb cycling offers a dietary strategy that supports optimal blood sugar regulation and metabolic health.

In addition to its metabolic benefits, carb cycling can also enhance physical performance and endurance in seniors. By strategically timing high-carb days to coincide with periods of increased physical activity or exercise, seniors can ensure they have an adequate supply of energy to fuel their workouts and promote recovery. Conversely, low-carb days promote fat oxidation and metabolic flexibility, which can improve endurance and stamina over time. This is particularly important for seniors looking to maintain an active lifestyle and preserve their independence as they age.

CHAPTER 1

NUTRITIONAL GUIDELINES FOR SENIOR CARB CYCLING

As individuals age, their nutritional needs undergo significant changes. One emerging approach to addressing these changing needs is senior carb cycling, a dietary strategy that involves alternating carbohydrate intake levels over a period of time. This method can be particularly beneficial for seniors, as it allows for better management of blood sugar levels, promotes weight loss, and supports overall health and well-being.

Carb cycling involves alternating between high-carb and low-carb days, with the goal of optimizing carbohydrate intake to match energy expenditure and activity levels. For seniors, this approach can help regulate blood sugar levels, which is crucial for preventing and managing conditions such as diabetes and insulin resistance. Additionally, carb cycling can support weight loss by promoting fat burning during low-carb days and providing energy for physical activity during high-carb days.

When implementing carb cycling for seniors, it's essential to consider individual dietary preferences, health status, and activity levels. Seniors should aim to consume complex carbohydrates such as whole grains, fruits, and vegetables during high-carb days, while limiting simple carbohydrates like refined sugars and processed foods. On low-carb days, emphasis should be placed on lean proteins, healthy fats, and non-starchy vegetables to promote satiety and support muscle maintenance.

It's also important for seniors to pay attention to portion sizes and meal timing when following a carb cycling approach. Eating smaller, more frequent meals throughout the day can help regulate blood sugar levels and prevent energy crashes, while also supporting metabolism and digestion. Additionally, timing carbohydrate intake around periods of physical activity can help optimize performance and recovery, particularly for seniors who engage in regular exercise or physical activity.

Incorporating senior carb cycling into a balanced diet can offer numerous benefits for older adults, including improved blood sugar control, weight management, and overall health and well-being. By carefully monitoring carbohydrate intake, portion sizes, and meal timing, seniors can optimize their nutritional intake and support healthy aging.

Macronutrient Breakdown for Seniors

As individuals age, their nutritional needs change, requiring adjustments to macronutrient intake to support overall health and well-being. Seniors often require different proportions of macronutrients compared to younger adults, with a greater emphasis on certain nutrients to support muscle maintenance, bone health, and cognitive function.

Protein is a critical macronutrient for seniors, playing a key role in muscle maintenance, repair, and immune function. As individuals age, muscle mass naturally declines, making adequate protein intake essential for preserving muscle mass and strength. Seniors should aim to include lean sources of protein such as poultry, fish, eggs, dairy products, legumes, and tofu in their diet to support muscle health and prevent age-related muscle loss.

Carbohydrates are another important macronutrient for seniors, providing energy for daily activities and supporting brain function. However, the type and amount of carbohydrates consumed should be carefully considered to prevent spikes in blood sugar levels and support overall health. Seniors should focus on consuming complex carbohydrates such as whole grains, fruits, and vegetables, while limiting simple carbohydrates like refined sugars and processed foods.

Fat is also a crucial macronutrient for seniors, providing essential fatty acids that support heart health, brain function, and hormone production. Seniors should aim to include healthy fats such as monounsaturated and polyunsaturated fats found in foods like nuts, seeds, avocados, and olive oil in their diet while limiting saturated and trans fats found in fried foods, baked goods, and processed snacks.

In addition to macronutrient proportions, seniors should also pay attention to meal timing and portion control to support optimal nutrition and overall health. Eating smaller, more frequent meals throughout the day can help regulate appetite, prevent overeating, and support digestion. Seniors should also strive to include a variety of nutrient-dense foods in their diet to ensure they are meeting their nutritional needs and supporting healthy aging.

By paying attention to macronutrient intake, meal timing, and portion control, seniors can optimize their nutritional intake and support overall health and well-being as they age.

Senior-Specific Nutritional Needs

As individuals age, their nutritional needs change, requiring adjustments to dietary intake to support optimal health and well-being. Seniors have unique nutritional needs influenced by factors such as changes in metabolism, decreased appetite, dental health issues, and chronic conditions. Understanding these specific nutritional needs is essential for promoting healthy aging and preventing age-related diseases.

One of the key nutritional needs for seniors is adequate protein intake to support muscle maintenance and repair. Age-related muscle loss, known as sarcopenia, is a common concern among older adults and can lead to decreased strength, mobility, and independence. Seniors should aim to include protein-rich foods such as lean meats, poultry, fish, eggs, dairy products, legumes, and tofu in their diet to support muscle health and prevent sarcopenia.

Calcium and vitamin D are also important nutrients for seniors, particularly for maintaining bone health and preventing osteoporosis. Seniors should aim to consume calcium-rich foods such as dairy products, leafy green vegetables, and fortified foods, along with vitamin D-rich foods such as fatty fish, egg yolks, and fortified dairy products. In some cases, supplementation may be necessary to ensure adequate intake of these essential nutrients.

Fiber is another important nutrient for seniors, supporting digestive health, regularity, and heart health. Seniors should aim to include fiber-rich foods such as whole grains, fruits, vegetables, legumes, and nuts in their diet to support optimal digestion and prevent constipation. Adequate hydration is also essential for supporting digestive health and preventing dehydration, particularly for seniors who may have decreased thirst sensation.

In addition to these specific nutritional needs, seniors should also pay attention to overall dietary patterns and lifestyle factors that can impact health and well-being. Eating a balanced diet rich in fruits, vegetables, whole grains, lean proteins, and healthy fats can help seniors meet their nutritional needs and support healthy aging. Regular physical activity, adequate sleep, and stress management are also important factors for maintaining optimal health and well-being as individuals age.

By understanding and addressing senior-specific nutritional needs, older adults can support healthy aging, maintain independence, and prevent age-related diseases.

Importance of Timing and Portion Control

When it comes to nutrition, timing and portion control are key factors that can significantly impact health and well-being, particularly for seniors. As individuals age, changes in metabolism, appetite, and digestion can affect how nutrients are absorbed and utilized by the body, making it important to pay attention to when and how much food is consumed.

One aspect of timing that is important for seniors is meal frequency and spacing. Eating smaller, more frequent meals throughout the day can help regulate appetite, prevent overeating, and support digestion, particularly for seniors who may have decreased appetite or difficulty eating larger meals. Additionally, spacing meals and snacks evenly throughout the day can help regulate blood sugar levels and prevent energy crashes.

Another aspect of timing to consider is the timing of carbohydrate intake, particularly for seniors who may be managing conditions such as diabetes or insulin resistance. Distributing carbohydrate intake evenly throughout the day and pairing carbohydrates with protein and healthy fats can help regulate blood sugar levels and prevent spikes and crashes. Additionally, timing carbohydrate intake around periods of physical activity can help optimize energy levels and support performance and recovery.

Portion control is another important aspect of nutrition for seniors, as changes in metabolism and activity levels can affect energy needs and calorie requirements. Seniors should aim to consume appropriate portion sizes based on their individual energy needs and activity levels, while also paying attention to hunger and satiety cues to prevent overeating. Using smaller plates, measuring serving sizes, and practicing mindful eating can help seniors control portion sizes and prevent excess calorie intake.

By paying attention to timing and portion control, seniors can optimize their nutritional intake, support overall health and well-being, and prevent age-related diseases. Incorporating these principles into a balanced diet and lifestyle can help seniors maintain independence, vitality, and quality of life as they age.

CHAPTER 2

HIGH CARB DAYS: RECIPES

BREAKFAST RECIPES

Sweet Potato Pancakes

Prep Time: 15 minutes

Cooking Time: 10 minutes

Serving Size: 2 pancakes

Ingredients:

- 1 cup mashed sweet potatoes
- 2 eggs
- 1/4 cup almond flour
- 1/2 tsp baking powder
- 1/2 tsp cinnamon
- 1/4 tsp nutmeg
- 1/4 cup milk of choice
- 1 tbsp coconut oil (for cooking)

Instructions:

1. In a bowl, mix together mashed sweet potatoes, eggs, almond flour, baking powder, cinnamon, nutmeg, and milk until well combined.

2. Heat coconut oil in a skillet over medium heat. Pour 1/4 cup of batter onto the skillet for each pancake.

3. Cook until bubbles form on the surface, then flip and cook until golden brown.

Nutritional Information (per serving):

- Calories: 215
- Protein: 9g
- Sodium: 110mg
- Potassium: 320mg
- Total Fat: 10g
- Saturated Fat: 4g
- Cholesterol: 186mg
- Carbohydrates: 25g
- Fiber: 4g
- Sugars: 6g

Apple Cinnamon Quinoa Breakfast Bowl

Prep Time: 5 minutes

Cooking Time: 15 minutes

Serving Size: 1 bowl

Ingredients:

- 1/2 cup cooked quinoa
- 1/2 apple, diced
- 1 tbsp almond butter
- 1/2 tsp cinnamon
- 1 tbsp honey or maple syrup

Instructions:

1. In a small saucepan, heat cooked quinoa and diced apple until warm.

2. Stir in almond butter, cinnamon, and honey or maple syrup until well combined.

3. Transfer to a bowland serve warm.

Nutritional Information (per serving):

- Calories: 280

- Protein: 7g

- Sodium: 5mg

- Potassium: 300mg

- Total Fat: 9g

- Saturated Fat: 1g

- Cholesterol: 0mg

- Carbohydrates: 45g

- Fiber: 6g

- Sugars: 18g

Blueberry Almond Butter Toast

Prep Time: 5 minutes

Cooking Time: 0 minutes

Serving Size: 1 slice of toast

Ingredients:

- 1 slice whole grain bread

- 1 tbsp almond butter

- 1/4 cup fresh blueberries

- 1 tsp honey

Instructions:

1. Toast the slice of bread until golden brown.

2. Spread almond butter evenly over the toast.

3. Top with fresh blueberries and drizzle with honey.

Nutritional Information (per serving):

- Calories: 220

- Protein: 7g

- Sodium: 220mg

- Potassium: 180mg

- Total Fat: 9g

- Saturated Fat: 1g

- Cholesterol: 0mg

- Carbohydrates: 30g

- Fiber: 5g

- Sugars: 10g

Coconut Chia Pudding

Prep Time: 5 minutes

Cooking Time: 0 minutes (plus chilling time)

Serving Size: 1 bowl

Ingredients:

- 1/4 cup chia seeds

- 1 cup coconut milk

- 1/2 tsp vanilla extract

- 1 tbsp maple syrup

- 1/4 cup sliced strawberries

- 1 tbsp shredded coconut (optional)

Instructions:

1. In a bowl, mix together chia seeds, coconut milk, vanilla extract, and maple syrup until well combined.

2. Cover and refrigerate for at least 2 hours or overnight, until thickened.

3. Serve chilled, topped with sliced strawberries and shredded coconut if desired.

Nutritional Information (per serving):

- Calories: 320
- Protein: 7g
- Sodium: 20mg
- Potassium: 210mg
- Total Fat: 25g
- Saturated Fat: 15g
- Cholesterol: 0mg
- Carbohydrates: 20g
- Fiber: 10g
- Sugars: 6g

Mixed Berry Smoothie Bowl

Prep Time: 5 minutes

Cooking Time: 0 minutes

Serving Size: 1 bowl

Ingredients:

- 1/2 cup mixed berries (such as strawberries, raspberries, and blueberries)

- 1/2 banana
- 1/4 cup Greek yogurt
- 1/4 cup almond milk
- 1 tbsp honey
- 1/4 cup granola

Instructions:

1. In a blender, combine mixed berries, banana, Greek yogurt, almond milk, and honey. Blend until smooth.
2. Pour into a bowl and top with granola.

Nutritional Information (per serving):

- Calories: 280
- Protein: 10g
- Sodium: 90mg
- Potassium: 320mg
- Total Fat: 6g
- Saturated Fat: 1g
- Cholesterol: 5mg
- Carbohydrates: 45g
- Fiber: 6g
- Sugars: 25g

Peanut Butter Banana Toast

Prep Time: 5 minutes

Cooking Time: 0 minutes

Serving Size: 1 slice of toast

Ingredients:

- 1 slice whole grain bread
- 2 tbsp peanut butter
- 1/2 banana, sliced
- 1 tsp honey

Instructions:

1. Toast the slice of bread until golden brown.
2. Spread peanut butter evenly over the toast.
3. Top with sliced banana and drizzle with honey.

Nutritional Information (per serving):

- Calories: 280
- Protein: 9g
- Sodium: 220mg
- Potassium: 360mg
- Total Fat: 14g
- Saturated Fat: 3g
- Cholesterol: 0mg
- Carbohydrates: 35g
- Fiber: 6g
- Sugars: 12g

Cinnamon Raisin Bagel with Cream Cheese

Prep Time: 5 minutes

Cooking Time: 0 minutes

Serving Size: 1 bagel

Ingredients:

- 1 cinnamon raisin bagel

- 2 tbsp cream cheese

Instructions:

1. Toast the cinnamon raisin bagel until lightly golden.

2. Spread cream cheese evenly over the bagel halves.

Nutritional Information (per serving):

- Calories: 320

- Protein: 9g

- Sodium: 380mg

- Potassium: 160mg

- Total Fat: 9g

- Saturated Fat: 5g

- Cholesterol: 30mg

- Carbohydrates: 50g

- Fiber: 3g

- Sugars: 10g

Banana Nut Muffins

Prep Time: 15 minutes

Cooking Time: 20 minutes

Serving Size: 1 muffin

Ingredients:

- 1 cup mashed bananas (about 2 bananas)

- 1/4 cup honey

- 1/4 cup coconut oil, melted

- 1 egg

- 1 tsp vanilla extract

- 1 1/2 cups almond flour
- 1/2 tsp baking soda
- 1/4 tsp salt
- 1/2 cup chopped walnuts

Instructions:

1. Preheat oven to 350°F. Line a muffin tin with paper liners.
2. In a large bowl, mix together mashed bananas, honey, coconut oil, egg, and vanilla extract until well combined.
3. Add almond flour, baking soda, and salt to the wet ingredients, stirring until just combined. Fold in chopped walnuts.
4. Divide the batter evenly among the muffin cups.
5. Bake for 20 minutes or until a toothpick inserted into the center comes out clean.

Nutritional Information (per serving):

- Calories: 280
- Protein: 7g
- Sodium: 120mg
- Potassium: 240mg
- Total Fat: 20g
- Saturated Fat: 7g
- Cholesterol: 30mg
- Carbohydrates: 22g
- Fiber: 4g
- Sugars: 12g

Chocolate Chip Banana Bread

Prep Time: 15 minutes

Cooking Time: 45 minutes

Serving Size: 1 slice

Ingredients:

- 3 ripe bananas, mashed
- 1/2 cup honey
- 1/4 cup coconut oil, melted
- 1 egg
- 1 tsp vanilla extract
- 1 1/2 cups whole wheat flour
- 1/2 tsp baking soda
- 1/4 tsp salt
- 1/2 cup dark chocolate chips

Instructions:

1. Preheat oven to 350°F. Grease a loaf pan with coconut oil or line with parchment paper.
2. In a large bowl, mix together mashed bananas, honey, coconut oil, egg, and vanilla extract until well combined.
3. Add whole wheat flour, baking soda, and salt to the wet ingredients, stirring until just combined. Fold in dark chocolate chips.
4. Pour the batter into the prepared loaf pan and smooth the top.
5. Bake for 45 minutes or until a toothpick inserted into the center comes out clean.

Nutritional Information (per serving):

- Calories: 230
- Protein: 4g
- Sodium: 110mg
- Potassium: 230mg
- Total Fat: 10g
- Saturated Fat: 7g
- Cholesterol: 20mg
- Carbohydrates: 33g
- Fiber: 4g
- Sugars: 18g

Banana Maple Oatmeal

Prep Time: 5 minutes

Cooking Time: 10 minutes

Serving Size: 1 bowl

Ingredients:

- 1/2 cup rolled oats
- 1 cup water
- 1 ripe banana, mashed
- 1 tbsp maple syrup
- 1/4 tsp cinnamon
- 1/4 cup chopped nuts (such as almonds or pecans)
- 1/4 cup milk of choice (optional)

Instructions:

1. In a saucepan, bring water to a boil. Stir in rolled oats and reduce heat to low. Cook for 5-7 minutes, stirring occasionally, until oats are tender.

2. Stir in mashed banana, maple syrup, and cinnamon until well combined.

3. Serve hot, topped with chopped nuts and a splash of milk if desired.

Nutritional Information (per serving):

- Calories: 320
- Protein: 9g
- Sodium: 10mg
- Potassium: 380mg
- Total Fat: 12g
- Saturated Fat: 1g
- Cholesterol: 0mg
- Carbohydrates: 50g
- Fiber: 7g
- Sugars: 15g

LUNCH RECIPES

Sweet Potato and Chickpea Buddha Bowl

Prep Time: 15 minutes

Cooking Time: 25 minutes

Serving Size: 1 bowl

Ingredients:

- 1 medium sweet potato, cubed
- 1/2 cup cooked quinoa
- 1/2 cup cooked chickpeas
- 1 cup mixed greens
- 1/4 avocado, sliced
- 1 tbsp olive oil
- 1/2 tsp paprika
- Salt and pepper to taste

Instructions:

1. Preheat oven to 400°F. Toss sweet potato cubes with olive oil, paprika, salt, and pepper. Roast in the oven for 20-25 minutes until tender.
2. Assemble the bowl by placing cooked quinoa, chickpeas, mixed greens, roasted sweet potato, and avocado slices in a bowl.
3. Drizzle with your favorite dressing and enjoy.

Nutritional Information (per serving):
- Calories: 450
- Protein: 12g
- Sodium: 250mg
- Potassium: 850mg

- Total Fat: 18g

- Saturated Fat: 2.5g

- Cholesterol: 0mg

- Carbohydrates: 65g

- Fiber: 12g

- Sugars: 8g

Quinoa Stuffed Bell Peppers

Prep Time: 15 minutes

Cooking Time: 40 minutes

Serving Size: 1 stuffed pepper

Ingredients:

- 2 large bell peppers

- 1 cup cooked quinoa

- 1/2 cup black beans, drained and rinsed

- 1/2 cup corn kernels

- 1/4 cup diced tomatoes

- 1/4 cup diced onion

- 1/4 cup shredded cheese

- 1 tsp chili powder

- 1/2 tsp cumin

- Salt and pepper to taste

Instructions:

1. Preheat oven to 375°F. Cut the tops off the bell peppers and remove the seeds and membranes.

2. In a bowl, mix together cooked quinoa, black beans, corn, diced tomatoes, diced onion, shredded cheese, chili powder, cumin, salt, and pepper.

3. Stuff the mixture into the bell peppers and place them in a baking dish.

4. Cover with foil and bake for 30 minutes. Remove foil and bake for an additional 10 minutes until peppers are tender and filling is heated through.

Nutritional Information (per serving):

- Calories: 320
- Protein: 15g
- Sodium: 280mg
- Potassium: 800mg
- Total Fat: 8g
- Saturated Fat: 3g
- Cholesterol: 15mg
- Carbohydrates: 50g
- Fiber: 10g
- Sugars: 8g

Vegetable Lentil Soup

Prep Time: 15 minutes

Cooking Time: 30 minutes

Serving Size: 1 bowl

Ingredients:

- 1 cup brown or green lentils, rinsed

- 4 cups vegetable broth
- 1 onion, diced
- 2 carrots, diced
- 2 celery stalks, diced
- 2 cloves garlic, minced
- 1 tsp dried thyme
- 1 tsp dried rosemary
- Salt and pepper to taste
- 2 tbsp olive oil

Instructions:

1. Heat olive oil in a large pot over medium heat. Add diced onion, carrots, celery, and garlic. Cook until vegetables are tender, about 5-7 minutes.

2. Add lentils, vegetable broth, dried thyme, dried rosemary, salt, and pepper to the pot. Bring to a boil, then reduce heat and simmer for 20-25 minutes until lentils are cooked through.

3. Taste and adjust seasoning if needed. Serve hot.

Nutritional Information (per serving):

- Calories: 280
- Protein: 15g
- Sodium: 750mg
- Potassium: 650mg
- Total Fat: 6g
- Saturated Fat: 1g
- Cholesterol: 0mg
- Carbohydrates: 40g

- Fiber: 15g
- Sugars: 5g

Mediterranean Chickpea Salad

Prep Time: 15 minutes

Cooking Time: 0 minutes

Serving Size: 1 bowl

Ingredients:

- 1 can chickpeas, drained and rinsed
- 1 cucumber, diced
- 1 bell pepper, diced
- 1/4 cup red onion, thinly sliced
- 1/4 cup Kalamata olives, pitted and sliced
- 1/4 cup crumbled feta cheese
- 2 tbsp olive oil
- 1 tbsp lemon juice
- 1 tsp dried oregano
- Salt and pepper to taste

Instructions:

1. In a large bowl, combine chickpeas, diced cucumber, diced bell pepper, sliced red onion, sliced Kalamata olives, and crumbled feta cheese.

2. In a small bowl, whisk together olive oil, lemon juice, dried oregano, salt, and pepper.

3. Pour dressing over salad and toss until well coated. Serve chilled.

Nutritional Information (per serving):

- Calories: 320

- Protein: 12g

- Sodium: 480mg

- Potassium: 600mg

- Total Fat: 15g

- Saturated Fat: 3g

- Cholesterol: 10mg

- Carbohydrates: 35g

- Fiber: 10g

- Sugars: 5g

Pasta Primavera

Prep Time: 10 minutes

Cooking Time: 15 minutes

Serving Size: 1 plate

Ingredients:

- 2 cups cooked pasta (such as whole wheat or gluten-free)

- 1 cup mixed vegetables (such as bell peppers, broccoli, carrots, and peas)

- 1/4 cup cherry tomatoes, halved

- 2 cloves garlic, minced

- 2 tbsp olive oil

- 1/4 cup grated Parmesan cheese

- Salt and pepper to taste

Instructions:

1. Cook pasta according to package instructions. Drain and set aside.

2. In a large skillet, heat olive oil over medium heat. Add minced garlic and cook until fragrant, about 1 minute.

3. Add mixed vegetables to the skillet and cook until tender, about 5-7 minutes.

4. Add cooked pasta and cherry tomatoes to the skillet. Toss until well combined and heated through.

5. Season with salt and pepper, then sprinkle grated Parmesan cheese on top before serving.

Nutritional Information (per serving):

- Calories: 380
- Protein: 12g
- Sodium: 200mg
- Potassium: 350mg
- Total Fat: 10g
- Saturated Fat: 2g
- Cholesterol: 5mg
- Carbohydrates: 60g
- Fiber: 8g
- Sugars: 5g

Vegetarian Chili

Prep Time: 15 minutes

Cooking Time: 30 minutes

Serving Size: 1 bowl

Ingredients:

- 1 can black beans, drained and rinsed
- 1 can kidney beans, drained and rinsed
- 1 can diced tomatoes
- 1 onion, diced
- 1 bell pepper, diced
- 2 cloves garlic, minced
- 2 tbsp olive oil
- 2 tbsp chili powder
- 1 tsp cumin
- 1/2 tsp paprika
- Salt and pepper to taste

Instructions:

1. In a large pot, heat olive oil over medium heat. Add diced onion, diced bell pepper, and minced garlic. Cook until vegetables are tender, about 5-7 minutes.

2. Add chili powder, cumin, paprika, salt, and pepper to the pot. Stir until vegetables are coated with spices.

3. Add black beans, kidney beans, and diced tomatoes to the pot. Stir to combine.

4. Bring chili to a simmer and let cook for 20-25 minutes, stirring occasionally.

5. Taste and adjust seasoning if needed. Serve hot.

Nutritional Information (per serving):

- Calories: 320
- Protein: 15g

- Sodium: 600mg

- Potassium: 850mg

- Total Fat: 10g

- Saturated Fat: 1.5g

- Cholesterol: 0mg

- Carbohydrates: 45g

- Fiber: 15g

- Sugars: 8g

Vegetable Stir-Fry with Tofu

Prep Time: 15 minutes

Cooking Time: 15 minutes

Serving Size: 1 plate

Ingredients: 1 block firm tofu, pressed and cubed

- 2 cups mixed vegetables (such as bell peppers, broccoli, snap peas, and carrots)

- 2 cloves garlic, minced

- 1 tbsp ginger, minced

- 2 tbsp soy sauce

- 1 tbsp hoisin sauce

- 1 tbsp sesame oil

- Cooked rice or quinoa for serving

Instructions:

1. Heat sesame oil in a large skillet or wok over medium-high heat. Add minced garlic and ginger, and cook until fragrant, about 1 minute.

2. Add cubed tofu to the skillet and cook until golden brown on all sides, about 5-7 minutes.

3. Add mixed vegetables to the skillet and stir-fry until tender-crisp, about 3-5 minutes.

4. Stir in soy sauce and hoisin sauce, and toss until everything is well coated.

5. Serve stir-fry hot over cooked rice or quinoa.

Nutritional Information (per serving):

- Calories: 380
- Protein: 25g
- Sodium: 800mg
- Potassium: 700mg
- Total Fat: 15g
- Saturated Fat: 2.5g
- Cholesterol: 0mg
- Carbohydrates: 45g
- Fiber: 8g
- Sugars: 8g

Mushroom and Spinach Quesadillas

Prep Time: 10 minutes

Cooking Time: 10 minutes

Serving Size: 1 quesadilla

Ingredients:

- 2 large whole wheat tortillas
- 1 cup sliced mushrooms
- 2 cups baby spinach

- 1/2 cup shredded cheese (such as cheddar or Monterey Jack)
- 1/4 cup salsa
- Cooking spray or butter for cooking

Instructions:

1. Heat a skillet over medium heat and coat with cooking spray or butter.
2. Place one tortilla in the skillet and sprinkle half of the shredded cheese over it.
3. Layer sliced mushrooms and baby spinach on top of the cheese.
4. Sprinkle remaining shredded cheese over the vegetables and top with the second tortilla.
5. Cook until the bottom tortilla is golden brown and the cheese is melted, about 3-4 minutes. Carefully flip the quesadilla and cook the other side until golden brown.
6. Remove from skillet, cut into wedges, and serve hot with salsa.

Nutritional Information (per serving):

- Calories: 350
- Protein: 15g
- Sodium: 750mg
- Potassium: 450mg
- Total Fat: 15g
- Saturated Fat: 6g
- Cholesterol: 30mg
- Carbohydrates: 40g
- Fiber: 8g
- Sugars: 5g

Roasted Vegetable and Hummus Wrap

Prep Time: 15 minutes

Cooking Time: 25 minutes

Serving Size: 1 wrap

Ingredients:

- 1 whole wheat tortilla
- 1/4 cup hummus
- 1/2 cup roasted vegetables (such as bell peppers, zucchini, eggplant, and onions)
- 1/4 cup mixed greens
- 1/4 avocado, sliced
- 1 tbsp balsamic glaze

Instructions:

1. Preheat oven to 400°F. Toss sliced vegetables with olive oil, salt, and pepper, and roast in the oven for 20-25 minutes until tender.
2. Spread hummus evenly over the whole wheat tortilla.
3. Layer roasted vegetables, mixed greens, and sliced avocado on top of the hummus.
4. Drizzle with balsamic glaze.
5. Roll up the tortilla tightly, slice in half, and serve.

Nutritional Information (per serving):

- Calories: 320
- Protein: 8g
- Sodium: 450mg
- Potassium: 600mg

- Total Fat: 15g

- Saturated Fat: 2g

- Cholesterol: 0mg

- Carbohydrates: 40g

- Fiber: 10g

- Sugars: 5g

Lentil and Vegetable Curry

Prep Time: 15 minutes

Cooking Time: 30 minutes

Serving Size: 1 bowl

Ingredients: 1 cup brown or green lentils, rinsed

- 2 cups vegetable broth, 1 onion, diced

- 2 cloves garlic, minced

- 1 bell pepper, diced

- 1 carrot, diced

- 1 zucchini, diced

- 1 can diced tomatoes

- 1 can coconut milk

- 2 tbsp curry powder

- 1 tsp turmeric

- Salt and pepper to taste

- 2 tbsp olive oil

Instructions:

1. Heat olive oil in a large pot over medium heat. Add diced onion and minced garlic, and cook until softened, about 5 minutes.

2. Add diced bell pepper, carrot, and zucchini to the pot. Cook until vegetables are tender, about 5-7 minutes.

3. Stir in curry powder and turmeric, and cook for 1 minute until fragrant.

4. Add rinsed lentils, vegetable broth, diced tomatoes, and coconut milk to the pot. Bring to a boil, then reduce heat and simmer for 20-25 minutes until lentils are cooked through.

5. Taste and adjust seasoning if needed. Serve hot over cooked rice or quinoa.

Nutritional Information (per serving):

- Calories: 380
- Protein: 15g
- Sodium: 750mg
- Potassium: 800mg
- Total Fat: 15g
- Saturated Fat: 8g
- Cholesterol: 0mg
- Carbohydrates: 50g
- Fiber: 15g
- Sugars: 8g

DINNER RECIPES

Sweet Potato and Lentil Shepherd's Pie

Prep Time: 20 minutes

Cooking Time: 40 minutes

Serving Size: 1 slice

Ingredients:

- 2 large sweet potatoes, peeled and diced
- 1 cup brown lentils, cooked
- 1 onion, diced
- 2 cloves garlic, minced
- 1 carrot, diced
- 1 celery stalk, diced
- 1 cup frozen peas
- 1 cup vegetable broth
- 2 tbsp tomato paste
- 1 tsp dried thyme
- Salt and pepper to taste
- 2 tbsp olive oil

Instructions:

1. Preheat oven to 375°F.
2. In a pot, boil sweet potatoes until tender. Drain and mash with a fork until smooth.
3. In a separate pot, heat olive oil over medium heat. Add diced onion, minced garlic, diced carrot, and diced celery. Cook until softened, about 5-7 minutes.

4. Add cooked lentils, frozen peas, vegetable broth, tomato paste, dried thyme, salt, and pepper to the pot. Stir well and simmer for 10-15 minutes until the mixture thickens.

5. Transfer the lentil mixture to a baking dish. Spread mashed sweet potatoes evenly over the top.

6. Bake in the preheated oven for 20-25 minutes until the sweet potatoes are golden brown.

7. Serve hot.

Nutritional Information (per serving):

- Calories: 320
- Protein: 10g
- Sodium: 450mg
- Potassium: 700mg
- Total Fat: 10g
- Saturated Fat: 1.5g
- Cholesterol: 0mg
- Carbohydrates: 50g
- Fiber: 10g
- Sugars: 8g

Chickpea and Vegetable Stir-Fry

Prep Time: 15 minutes

Cooking Time: 15 minutes

Serving Size: 1 plate

Ingredients:

- 1 can chickpeas, drained and rinsed
- 2 cups mixed vegetables (such as bell peppers, broccoli, snap peas, and carrots)
- 2 cloves garlic, minced
- 1 tbsp ginger, minced
- 2 tbsp soy sauce
- 1 tbsp hoisin sauce
- 1 tbsp sesame oil
- Cooked rice for serving

Instructions:

1. Heat sesame oil in a large skillet or wok over medium-high heat. Add minced garlic and ginger, and cook until fragrant, about 1 minute.
2. Add mixed vegetables to the skillet and stir-fry until tender-crisp, about 3-5 minutes.
3. Stir in chickpeas, soy sauce, and hoisin sauce, and toss until everything is well coated and heated through.
4. Serve stir-fry hot over cooked rice.

Nutritional Information (per serving):

- Calories: 380
- Protein: 15g
- Sodium: 800mg
- Potassium: 700mg
- Total Fat: 15g

- Saturated Fat: 2.5g
- Cholesterol: 0mg
- Carbohydrates: 45g
- Fiber: 8g
- Sugars: 5g

Vegetarian Chili

Prep Time: 15 minutes

Cooking Time: 30 minutes

Serving Size: 1 bowl

Ingredients:

- 1 can black beans, drained and rinsed
- 1 can kidney beans, drained and rinsed
- 1 can diced tomatoes
- 1 onion, diced
- 2 cloves garlic, minced
- 1 bell pepper, diced
- 1 carrot, diced
- 1 zucchini, diced
- 2 cups vegetable broth
- 2 tbsp chili powder
- 1 tsp ground cumin
- Salt and pepper to taste
- 2 tbsp olive oil

Instructions:

1. Heat olive oil in a large pot over medium heat. Add diced onion and minced garlic, and cook until softened, about 5 minutes.

2. Add diced bell pepper, carrot, and zucchini to the pot. Cook until vegetables are tender, about 5-7 minutes.

3. Stir in chili powder and ground cumin, and cook for 1 minute until fragrant.

4. Add black beans, kidney beans, diced tomatoes, and vegetable broth to the pot. Bring to a boil, then reduce heat and simmer for 20-25 minutes until flavors are combined and chili has thickened.

5. Taste and adjust seasoning if needed. Serve hot.

Nutritional Information (per serving):

- Calories: 320
- Protein: 15g
- Sodium: 750mg
- Potassium: 800mg
- Total Fat: 15g
- Saturated Fat: 2g
- Cholesterol: 0mg
- Carbohydrates: 45g
- Fiber: 12g
- Sugars: 8g

Quinoa Stuffed Bell Peppers

Prep Time: 20 minutes

Cooking Time: 30 minutes

Serving Size: 1 stuffed pepper

Ingredients:

- 4 large bell peppers, halved and seeds removed
- 1 cup quinoa, cooked
- 1 can black beans, drained and rinsed
- 1 cup corn kernels
- 1 cup diced tomatoes
- 1/2 cup diced red onion
- 1/2 cup shredded cheese (such as cheddar or Monterey Jack)
- 2 tbsp chopped cilantro
- 1 tsp ground cumin
- Salt and pepper to taste
- Cooking spray or olive oil for cooking

Instructions:

1. Preheat oven to 375°F. Lightly coat a baking dish with cooking spray or olive oil.
2. In a large bowl, combine cooked quinoa, black beans, corn kernels, diced tomatoes, diced red onion, shredded cheese, chopped cilantro, ground cumin, salt, and pepper.
3. Spoon quinoa mixture into each halved bell pepper, pressing down gently to pack the filling.
4. Place stuffed bell peppers in the prepared baking dish. Cover with aluminum foil and bake for 25 minutes.
5. Remove foil and bake for an additional 5-10 minutes until peppers are tender and filling is heated through.
6. Serve hot.

Nutritional Information (per serving):

- Calories: 350
- Protein: 15g
- Sodium: 550mg
- Potassium: 700mg
- Total Fat: 10g
- Saturated Fat: 3g
- Cholesterol: 15mg
- Carbohydrates: 55g
- Fiber: 12g
- Sugars: 8g

Vegetable and Chickpea Coconut Curry

Prep Time: 15 minutes

Cooking Time: 25 minutes

Serving Size: 1 bowl

Ingredients:

- 1 can chickpeas, drained and rinsed
- 1 onion, diced
- 2 cloves garlic, minced
- 1 bell pepper, diced
- 1 carrot, diced
- 1 zucchini, diced
- 1 cup coconut milk
- 1 cup vegetable broth
- 2 tbsp curry powder

- 1 tsp ground turmeric
- 1/2 tsp ground ginger
- Salt and pepper to taste
- 2 tbsp olive oil

Instructions:

1. Heat olive oil in a large pot over medium heat. Add diced onion and minced garlic, and cook until softened, about 5 minutes.

2. Add diced bell pepper, carrot, and zucchini to the pot. Cook until vegetables are tender, about 5-7 minutes.

3. Stir in curry powder, ground turmeric, and ground ginger, and cook for 1 minute until fragrant.

4. Add chickpeas, coconut milk, and vegetable broth to the pot. Bring to a simmer and cook for 10-15 minutes until flavors are combined and curry has thickened.

5. Taste and adjust seasoning if needed. Serve hot over cooked rice.

Nutritional Information (per serving):

- Calories: 380
- Protein: 15g
- Sodium: 650mg
- Potassium: 750mg
- Total Fat: 15g
- Saturated Fat: 5g
- Cholesterol: 0mg
- Carbohydrates: 45g
- Fiber: 10g
- Sugars: 8g

Mushroom and Spinach Pasta

Prep Time: 15 minutes

Cooking Time: 20 minutes

Serving Size: 1 plate

Ingredients:

- 2 cups whole wheat pasta
- 2 cups sliced mushrooms
- 2 cups baby spinach
- 2 cloves garlic, minced
- 1/4 cup diced onion
- 1/4 cup grated Parmesan cheese
- 2 tbsp olive oil
- Salt and pepper to taste

Instructions:

1. Cook pasta according to package instructions. Drain and set aside.
2. In a large skillet, heat olive oil over medium heat. Add minced garlic and diced onion, and cook until softened, about 2-3 minutes.
3. Add sliced mushrooms to the skillet and cook until golden brown, about 5 minutes.
4. Stir in baby spinach and cooked pasta, and cook until spinach is wilted, about 2-3 minutes.
5. Remove from heat and stir in grated Parmesan cheese. Season with salt and pepper to taste.
6. Serve hot.

Nutritional Information (per serving):

- Calories: 350
- Protein: 12g
- Sodium: 350mg
- Potassium: 500mg
- Total Fat: 10g
- Saturated Fat: 2g
- Cholesterol: 5mg
- Carbohydrates: 50g
- Fiber: 8g
- Sugars: 5g

Vegetable and Tofu Stir-Fry with Rice Noodles

Prep Time: 15 minutes

Cooking Time: 15 minutes

Serving Size: 1 plate

Ingredients:

- 6 oz rice noodles
- 1 block firm tofu, cubed
- 2 cups mixed vegetables (such as bell peppers, broccoli, snap peas, and carrots)
- 2 cloves garlic, minced
- 1 tbsp ginger, minced
- 2 tbsp soy sauce
- 1 tbsp hoisin sauce
- 1 tbsp sesame oil

- Salt and pepper to taste

Instructions:

1. Cook rice noodles according to package instructions. Drain and set aside.

2. Heat sesame oil in a large skillet or wok over medium-high heat. Add minced garlic and ginger, and cook until fragrant, about 1 minute.

3. Add cubed tofu to the skillet and cook until golden brown on all sides, about 5-7 minutes.

4. Add mixed vegetables to the skillet and stir-fry until tender-crisp, about 3-5 minutes.

5. Stir in soy sauce and hoisin sauce, and toss until everything is well coated.

6. Serve stir-fry hot over cooked rice noodles.

Nutritional Information (per serving):

- Calories: 380
- Protein: 20g
- Sodium: 800mg
- Potassium: 700mg
- Total Fat: 15g
- Saturated Fat: 2.5g
- Cholesterol: 0mg
- Carbohydrates: 45g
- Fiber: 8g
- Sugars: 5g

Butternut Squash and Chickpea Curry

Prep Time: 20 minutes

Cooking Time: 30 minutes

Serving Size: 1 bowl

Ingredients:

- 2 cups cubed butternut squash

- 1 can chickpeas, drained and rinsed

- 1 onion, diced

- 2 cloves garlic, minced

- 1 tbsp ginger, minced

- 1 can coconut milk

- 1 cup vegetable broth

- 2 tbsp curry powder

- 1 tsp ground turmeric

- Salt and pepper to taste

- 2 tbsp olive oil

Instructions:

1. Heat olive oil in a large pot over medium heat. Add diced onion, minced garlic, and minced ginger, and cook until softened, about 5 minutes.

2. Add cubed butternut squash to the pot and cook until slightly softened, about 5 minutes.

3. Stir in curry powder and ground turmeric, and cook for 1 minute until fragrant.

4. Add chickpeas, coconut milk, and vegetable broth to the pot. Bring to a simmer and cook for 15-20 minutes until squash is tender and curry has thickened.

5. Taste and adjust seasoning if needed. Serve hot over cooked rice.

Nutritional Information (per serving):

- Calories: 380

- Protein: 15g

- Sodium: 650mg

- Potassium: 800mg

- Total Fat: 15g

- Saturated Fat: 5g

- Cholesterol: 0mg

- Carbohydrates: 55g

- Fiber: 12g

- Sugars: 8g

Tomato and Basil Pasta

Prep Time: 10 minutes

Cooking Time: 20 minutes

Serving Size: 1 plate

Ingredients:

- 2 cups whole wheat pasta
- 2 cups cherry tomatoes, halved
- 2 cloves garlic, minced
- 1/4 cup fresh basil leaves, chopped
- 2 tbsp olive oil
- Salt and pepper to taste

Instructions:

1. Cook pasta according to package instructions. Drain and set aside.
2. In a large skillet, heat olive oil over medium heat. Add minced garlic and cook until fragrant, about 1 minute.
3. Add cherry tomatoes to the skillet and cook until softened, about 5-7 minutes.
4. Stir in cooked pasta and chopped basil leaves, and toss until everything is well combined.
5. Season with salt and pepper to taste. Serve hot.

Nutritional Information (per serving):

- Calories: 320
- Protein: 10g
- Sodium: 350mg
- Potassium: 450mg
- Total Fat: 10g
- Saturated Fat: 1.5g
- Cholesterol: 0mg
- Carbohydrates: 45g
- Fiber: 8g

- Sugars: 5g

Vegetable and Lentil Soup

Prep Time: 15 minutes

Cooking Time: 30 minutes

Serving Size: 1 bowl

Ingredients:

- 1 cup brown lentils, cooked
- 2 carrots, diced
- 2 celery stalks, diced
- 1 onion, diced
- 2 cloves garlic, minced
- 4 cups vegetable broth
- 1 can diced tomatoes
- 1 tsp dried thyme
- 1 tsp dried oregano
- Salt and pepper to taste
- 2 tbsp olive oil

Instructions:

1. Heat olive oil in a large pot over medium heat. Add diced onion and minced garlic, and cook until softened, about 5 minutes.

2. Add diced carrots and diced celery to the pot. Cook until vegetables are slightly softened, about 5 minutes.

3. Stir in cooked brown lentils, vegetable broth, diced tomatoes, dried thyme, dried oregano, salt, and pepper. Bring to a boil,

then reduce heat and simmer for 20-25 minutes until flavors
are combined.

4. Taste and adjust seasoning if needed. Serve hot.

Nutritional Information (per serving):

- Calories: 280

- Protein: 10g

- Sodium: 750mg

- Potassium: 650mg

- Total Fat: 10g

- Saturated Fat: 1.5g

- Cholesterol: 0mg

- Carbohydrates: 40g

- Fiber: 10g

- Sugars: 5g

SNACKS RECIPES

Sweet Potato Toast with Almond Butter and Banana

Prep Time: 5 minutes

Cooking Time: 10 minutes

Serving Size: 2 slices

Ingredients:

- 1 large sweet potato, sliced lengthwise into 1/4 inch thick slices
- 2 tbsp almond butter
- 1 ripe banana, thinly sliced
- Optional toppings: honey, cinnamon

Instructions:

1. Preheat oven to 400°F. Place sweet potato slices on a baking sheet lined with parchment paper.
2. Bake sweet potato slices for 10-15 minutes until tender.
3. Remove sweet potato slices from the oven and let cool slightly.
4. Spread almond butter evenly on each sweet potato slice.
5. Top with thinly sliced banana. Drizzle with honey and sprinkle with cinnamon if desired.
6. Serve immediately and enjoy!

Nutritional Information (per serving):

- Calories: 180
- Protein: 4g
- Sodium: 80mg
- Potassium: 420mg

- Total Fat: 6g
- Saturated Fat: 0.5g
- Cholesterol: 0mg
- Carbohydrates: 30g
- Fiber: 5g
- Sugars: 10g

Energy Bites with Oats and Dates

Prep Time: 10 minutes

Cooking Time: 0 minutes (no-bake)

Serving Size: 2 bites

Ingredients:

- 1 cup rolled oats
- 1/2 cup medjool dates, pitted
- 1/4 cup almond butter
- 2 tbsp honey or maple syrup
- 1/4 cup chopped nuts (such as almonds or walnuts)
- 1/4 cup shredded coconut (optional)
- 1 tsp vanilla extract
- Pinch of salt

Instructions:

1. In a food processor, combine rolled oats, pitted dates, almond butter, honey or maple syrup, chopped nuts, shredded coconut (if using), vanilla extract, and a pinch of salt.

2. Pulse until the mixture comes together and forms a sticky dough.

3. Roll the dough into small balls, about 1 inch in diameter.

4. Place the energy bites on a plate or baking sheet lined with parchment paper.

5. Refrigerate for at least 30 minutes to firm up.

6. Once firm, store the energy bites in an airtight container in the refrigerator for up to one week.

7. Enjoy as a quick and nutritious snack!

Nutritional Information (per serving):

- Calories: 150
- Protein: 4g
- Sodium: 20mg
- Potassium: 180mg
- Total Fat: 7g
- Saturated Fat: 1g
- Cholesterol: 0mg
- Carbohydrates: 20g
- Fiber: 3g
- Sugars: 10g

Hummus and Veggie Dip Platter

Prep Time: 10 minutes

Cooking Time: 0 minutes

Serving Size: 1/4 cup hummus with assorted veggies

Ingredients:

- 1 cup chickpeas, drained and rinsed
- 2 tbsp tahini
- 2 tbsp lemon juice

- 1 clove garlic, minced
- 2 tbsp olive oil
- Salt and pepper to taste
- Assorted veggies for dipping (carrot sticks, cucumber slices, bell pepper strips, cherry tomatoes)

Instructions:

1. In a food processor, combine chickpeas, tahini, lemon juice, minced garlic, olive oil, salt, and pepper.
2. Blend until smooth and creamy, adding a splash of water if needed to achieve desired consistency.
3. Transfer hummus to a serving bowl and arrange assorted veggies on a platter.
4. Serve hummus with veggies for dipping.
5. Enjoy this healthy and satisfying snack!

Nutritional Information (per serving):

- Calories: 120
- Protein: 4g
- Sodium: 120mg
- Potassium: 180mg
- Total Fat: 7g
- Saturated Fat: 1g
- Cholesterol: 0mg
- Carbohydrates: 12g
- Fiber: 3g
- Sugars: 2g

Banana Oatmeal Cookies

Prep Time: 10 minutes

Cooking Time: 15 minutes

Serving Size: 2 cookies

Ingredients:

- 2 ripe bananas, mashed
- 1 cup rolled oats
- 1/4 cup raisins or chocolate chips
- 1/4 cup chopped nuts (such as walnuts or pecans)
- 1 tsp vanilla extract
- Pinch of cinnamon (optional)

Instructions:

1. Preheat oven to 350°F and line a baking sheet with parchment paper.
2. In a mixing bowl, combine mashed bananas, rolled oats, raisins or chocolate chips, chopped nuts, vanilla extract, and a pinch of cinnamon (if using). Mix until well combined.
3. Drop spoonfuls of the cookie dough onto the prepared baking sheet, spacing them apart.
4. Flatten each cookie slightly with the back of a spoon or fork.
5. Bake in the preheated oven for 12-15 minutes until golden brown.
6. Remove from the oven and let cool on the baking sheet for 5 minutes before transferring to a wire rack to cool completely.
7. Enjoy these delicious and wholesome cookies as a snack!

Nutritional Information (per serving):

- Calories: 150
- Protein: 3g
- Sodium: 0mg
- Potassium: 200mg
- Total Fat: 5g
- Saturated Fat: 1g
- Cholesterol: 0mg
- Carbohydrates: 25g
- Fiber: 3g
- Sugars: 10g

Greek Yogurt Parfait with Berries and Granola

Prep Time: 5 minutes

Cooking Time: 0 minutes

Serving Size: 1 parfait

Ingredients:

- 1/2 cup Greek yogurt
- 1/4 cup mixed berries (such as strawberries, blueberries, raspberries)
- 1/4 cup granola
- Drizzle of honey (optional)

Instructions:

1. In a glass or serving bowl, layer Greek yogurt, mixed berries, and granola.

2. Repeat the layers until the ingredients are used up, ending with a layer of granola on top.

3. Drizzle with honey if desired.

4. Serve immediately and enjoy this refreshing and nutritious snack!

Nutritional Information (per serving):

- Calories: 200
- Protein: 10g
- Sodium: 40mg
- Potassium: 250mg
- Total Fat: 4g
- Saturated Fat: 0.5g
- Cholesterol: 5mg
- Carbohydrates: 30g
- Fiber: 3g
- Sugars: 15g

CHAPTER 3

LOW CARB DAYS: RECIPES

BREAKFAST RECIPES

Spinach and Feta Crustless Quiche

Prep Time: 10 minutes

Cooking Time: 30 minutes

Serving Size: 1 slice

Ingredients:

- 4 large eggs
- 1 cup spinach, chopped
- 1/2 cup feta cheese, crumbled
- 1/4 cup diced onion
- 1/4 cup diced bell pepper
- 1/4 cup diced tomatoes
- Salt and pepper to taste
- Cooking spray or olive oil for greasing

Instructions:

1. Preheat oven to 350°F and grease a pie dish with cooking spray or olive oil.

2. In a mixing bowl, whisk together eggs, chopped spinach, crumbled feta cheese, diced onion, diced bell pepper, diced tomatoes, salt, and pepper.

3. Pour the egg mixture into the prepared pie dish.

4. Bake for 25-30 minutes until the quiche is set and slightly golden on top.

5. Let cool for a few minutes before slicing and serving.

Nutritional Information (per serving):

- Calories: 120
- Protein: 9g
- Sodium: 300mg
- Potassium: 180mg
- Total Fat: 7g
- Saturated Fat: 3g
- Cholesterol: 190mg
- Carbohydrates: 4g
- Fiber: 1g
- Sugars: 2g

Egg and Avocado Breakfast Wrap

Prep time: 5 minutes

Cooking Time: 30 minutes

Serving Size: 1 wrap

Ingredients:

- 2 large eggs
- 1 whole wheat or low-carb tortilla
- 1/2 avocado, sliced
- Handful of baby spinach leaves
- Salt and pepper to taste
- Cooking spray or olive oil for cooking

Instructions:

1. In a small skillet, heat cooking spray or olive oil over medium heat.

2. Crack the eggs into the skillet and cook to desired doneness (scrambled, fried, or poached).

3. Season eggs with salt and pepper.

4. Warm the tortilla in the skillet for a few seconds on each side.

5. Place the tortilla on a plate and layer with cooked eggs, sliced avocado, and baby spinach leaves.

6. Roll up the tortilla into a wrap and serve immediately.

Nutritional Information (per serving):

- Calories: 300
- Protein: 14g
- Sodium: 350mg
- Potassium: 400mg
- Total Fat: 18g
- Saturated Fat: 4g
- Cholesterol: 370mg
- Carbohydrates: 24g
- Fiber: 8g
- Sugars: 1g

Greek Yogurt Parfait with Nuts and Berries

Prep Time: 5 minutes

Cooking Time: 0 minutes

Serving Size: 1 parfait

Ingredients:

- 1/2 cup Greek yogurt
- 1/4 cup mixed berries (such as strawberries, blueberries, raspberries)
- 2 tbsp chopped nuts (such as almonds, walnuts, or pecans)
- Drizzle of honey (optional)

Instructions:

1. In a glass or serving bowl, layer Greek yogurt, mixed berries, and chopped nuts.
2. Repeat the layers until the ingredients are used up.
3. Drizzle with honey if desired.
4. Serve immediately and enjoy this protein-packed breakfast!

Nutritional Information (per serving):

- Calories: 250
- Protein: 18g
- Sodium: 70mg
- Potassium: 320mg
- Total Fat: 12g
- Saturated Fat: 2g
- Cholesterol: 10mg
- Carbohydrates: 20g
- Fiber: 5g
- Sugars: 12g

Low-Carb Breakfast Casserole

Prep Time: 15 minutes

Cooking Time: 35 minutes

Serving Size: 1 slice

Ingredients:

- 6 large eggs
- 1/2 cup diced ham or cooked bacon
- 1/2 cup diced bell pepper
- 1/2 cup diced onion
- 1/2 cup shredded cheddar cheese
- 1/4 cup almond milk or heavy cream
- Salt and pepper to taste
- Cooking spray or olive oil for greasing

Instructions:

1. Preheat oven to 375°F and grease a baking dish with cooking spray or olive oil.
2. In a mixing bowl, whisk together eggs, diced ham or bacon, diced bell pepper, diced onion, shredded cheddar cheese, almond milk or heavy cream, salt, and pepper.
3. Pour the egg mixture into the prepared baking dish.
4. Bake for 30-35 minutes until the casserole is set and golden on top.
5. Let cool for a few minutes before slicing and serving.

Nutritional Information (per serving):

- Calories: 200

- Protein: 15g
- Sodium: 400mg
- Potassium: 200mg
- Total Fat: 12g
- Saturated Fat: 5g
- Cholesterol: 270mg
- Carbohydrates: 5g
- Fiber: 1g
- Sugars: 2g

Zucchini and Cheese Omelette

Prep Time: 10 minutes

Cooking Time: 10 minutes

Serving Size: 1 omelette

Ingredients:

- 2 large eggs
- 1/2 cup grated zucchini
- 1/4 cup shredded cheese (such as cheddar or mozzarella)
- 1/4 cup diced tomato
- Salt and pepper to taste
- Cooking spray or olive oil for cooking

Instructions:

1. In a mixing bowl, beat the eggs until well combined. Stir in grated zucchini, shredded cheese, diced tomato, salt, and pepper.

2. Heat cooking spray or olive oil in a non-stick skillet over medium heat.

3. Pour the egg mixture into the skillet and cook for 2-3 minutes until the edges start to set.

4. Use a spatula to lift the edges of the omelette and allow any uncooked egg to flow underneath.

5. Cook for an additional 2-3 minutes until the omelette is set and the bottom is golden brown.

6. Carefully fold the omelette in half and slide onto a plate.

7. Serve hot and enjoy!

Nutritional Information (per serving):

- Calories: 180
- Protein: 15g
- Sodium: 350mg
- Potassium: 250mg
- Total Fat: 10g
- Saturated Fat: 4g
- Cholesterol: 370mg
- Carbohydrates: 5g
- Fiber: 1g
- Sugars: 2g

Salmon and Avocado Breakfast Salad

Prep Time: 10 minutes

Cooking Time: 10 minutes

Serving Size: 1 salad

Ingredients:

- 4 oz smoked salmon

- 1/2 avocado, sliced

- 1 cup mixed salad greens (such as spinach, arugula, or kale)

- 1/4 cup cherry tomatoes, halved

- 1 tbsp extra virgin olive oil

- 1 tbsp lemon juice

- Salt and pepper to taste

Instructions:

1. In a large bowl, toss together mixed salad greens and cherry tomatoes.

2. Drizzle extra virgin olive oil and lemon juice over the salad. Season with salt and pepper to taste.

3. Arrange smoked salmon and sliced avocado on top of the salad.

4. Serve immediately and enjoy this refreshing and protein-rich breakfast!

Nutritional Information (per serving):

- Calories: 280

- Protein: 20g

- Sodium: 550mg

- Potassium: 600mg

- Total Fat: 18g

- Saturated Fat: 3g

- Cholesterol: 25mg

- Carbohydrates: 10g

- Fiber: 5g

- Sugars: 2g

Cottage Cheese and Berry Bowl

Prep Time: 5 minutes

Cooking Time: 20 minutes

Serving Size: 1 bowl

Ingredients:

- 1/2 cup low-fat cottage cheese
- 1/4 cup mixed berries (such as strawberries, blueberries, raspberries)
- 1 tbsp chopped nuts (such as almonds, walnuts, or pecans)
- Drizzle of honey (optional)

Instructions:

1. In a bowl, spoon low-fat cottage cheese.
2. Top with mixed berries and chopped nuts.
3. Drizzle with honey if desired.
4. Serve immediately and enjoy this protein-packed and nutritious breakfast!

Nutritional Information (per serving):

- Calories: 180
- Protein: 15g
- Sodium: 400mg
- Potassium: 200mg
- Total Fat: 8g
- Saturated Fat: 2g
- Cholesterol: 15mg
- Carbohydrates: 10g

- Fiber: 2g
- Sugars: 7g

Low-Carb Veggie and Cheese Frittata

Prep Time: 10 minutes

Cooking Time: 20 minutes

Serving Size: 1 slice

Ingredients:

- 6 large eggs
- 1 cup chopped mixed vegetables (such as bell peppers, mushrooms, spinach, onions)
- 1/2 cup shredded cheese (such as cheddar or mozzarella)
- 1/4 cup almond milk or heavy cream
- Salt and pepper to taste
- Cooking spray or olive oil for greasing

Instructions:

1. Preheat oven to 375°F and grease a pie dish with cooking spray or olive oil.
2. In a mixing bowl, whisk together eggs, chopped mixed vegetables, shredded cheese, almond milk or heavy cream, salt, and pepper.
3. Pour the egg mixture into the prepared pie dish.
4. Bake for 18-20 minutes until the frittata is set and slightly golden on top.
5. Let cool for a few minutes before slicing and serving.

Nutritional Information (per serving):

- Calories: 150

- Protein: 12g

- Sodium: 300mg

- Potassium: 200mg

- Total Fat: 9g

- Saturated Fat: 3.5g

- Cholesterol: 280mg

- Carbohydrates: 5g

- Fiber: 1g

- Sugars: 2g

Low-Carb Breakfast Smootzie

Prep Time: 5 minutes

Cooking Time: 20 minutes

Serving Size: 1 smoothie

Ingredients:

- 1/2 cup unsweetened almond milk

- 1/4 cup Greek yogurt

- 1/4 cup frozen berries (such as strawberries, blueberries, raspberries)

- 1/4 avocado

- 1 tbsp almond butter

- 1/2 tsp vanilla extract

- Ice cubes (optional)

Instructions:

1. In a blender, combine unsweetened almond milk, Greek yogurt, frozen berries, avocado, almond butter, vanilla extract, and ice cubes (if using).

2. Blend until smooth and creamy.

3. Pour into a glass and serve immediately.

Nutritional Information (per serving):

- Calories: 250
- Protein: 10g
- Sodium: 200mg
- Potassium: 400mg
- Total Fat: 18g
- Saturated Fat: 2g
- Cholesterol: 10mg
- Carbohydrates: 15g
- Fiber: 7g
- Sugars: 6g

Low-Carb Breakfast Egg Muffins

Prep Time: 10 minutes

Cooking Time: 20 minutes

Serving Size: 1 muffin

Ingredients:

- 6 large eggs
- 1/2 cup diced bell pepper
- 1/4 cup diced onion

- 1/4 cup diced tomatoes
- 1/4 cup shredded cheese (such as cheddar or mozzarella)
- Salt and pepper to taste
- Cooking spray or olive oil for greasing

Instructions:

1. Preheat oven to 350°F and grease a muffin tin with cooking spray or olive oil.

2. In a mixing bowl, whisk together eggs, diced bell pepper, diced onion, diced tomatoes, shredded cheese, salt, and pepper.

3. Pour the egg mixture evenly into the muffin cups, filling each about 3/4 full.

4. Bake for 18-20 minutes until the egg muffins are set and slightly golden on top.

5. Let cool for a few minutes before removing from the muffin tin.

Nutritional Information (per serving):

- Calories: 100
- Protein: 7g
- Sodium: 200mg
- Potassium: 150mg
- Total Fat: 6g
- Saturated Fat: 2g
- Cholesterol: 190mg
- Carbohydrates: 3g
- Fiber: 1g
- Sugars: 1g

LUNCH RECIPES

Grilled Chicken Caesar Salad

Prep Time: 15 minutes

Cooking Time: 15 minutes

Serving Size: 1 salad

Ingredients:

- 4 oz grilled chicken breast, sliced
- 2 cups romaine lettuce, chopped
- 1/4 cup cherry tomatoes, halved
- 1/4 cup cucumber, sliced
- 2 tbsp grated Parmesan cheese
- 2 tbsp Caesar dressing (look for a low-carb option)
- Salt and pepper to taste

Instructions:

1. Season the chicken breast with salt and pepper and grill until cooked through.
2. In a large bowl, combine the romaine lettuce, cherry tomatoes, and cucumber.
3. Add the sliced grilled chicken on top.
4. Sprinkle grated Parmesan cheese over the salad.
5. Drizzle Caesar dressing over the salad and toss to coat evenly.
6. Serve immediately as a delicious and satisfying low-carb lunch option.

Nutritional Information (per serving):

- Calories: 250

- Protein: 30g

- Sodium: 400mg

- Potassium: 500mg

- Total Fat: 10g

- Saturated Fat: 3g

- Cholesterol: 80mg

- Carbohydrates: 8g

- Fiber: 3g

- Sugars: 3g

Turkey and Avocado Lettuce Wraps

Prep Time: 10 minutes

Serving Size: 2 wraps

Ingredients:

- 4 large lettuce leaves (such as romaine or iceberg)

- 6 oz sliced turkey breast

- 1 avocado, sliced

- 1/4 cup shredded carrots

- 1/4 cup sliced bell peppers

- 2 tbsp hummus (choose a low-carb variety)

- Salt and pepper to tast

Instructions:

1. Lay out the lettuce leaves on a flat surface.

2. Spread 1 tablespoon of hummus onto each lettuce leaf.

3. Divide the sliced turkey, avocado, shredded carrots, and sliced bell peppers evenly among the lettuce leaves.

4. Season with salt and pepper to taste.

5. Roll up each lettuce leaf into a wrap and secure with toothpicks if needed.

6. Serve immediately as a refreshing and nutritious low-carb lunch option.

Nutritional Information (per serving):

- Calories: 280
- Protein: 25g
- Sodium: 400mg
- Potassium: 600mg
- Total Fat: 15g
- Saturated Fat: 2g
- Cholesterol: 40mg
- Carbohydrates: 10g
- Fiber: 6g
- Sugars: 2g

Zucchini Noodles with Pesto and Grilled Shrimp

Prep Time: 20 minutes

Cooking Time: 10 minutes

Serving Size: 1 serving

Ingredients:

- 1 medium zucchini, spiralized into noodles
- 6 large shrimp, peeled and deveined
- 2 tbsp pesto sauce (look for a low-carb option)
- 1 tbsp olive oil

- 1 clove garlic, minced
- Salt and pepper to taste

Instructions:

1. Heat olive oil in a skillet over medium heat.

2. Add minced garlic to the skillet and sauté until fragrant.

3. Add the spiralized zucchini noodles to the skillet and cook for 2-3 minutes until tender.

4. Season the shrimp with salt and pepper and grill until cooked through.

5. Toss the cooked zucchini noodles with pesto sauce until evenly coated.

6. Serve the zucchini noodles topped with grilled shrimp for a light and flavorful low-carb lunch.

Nutritional Information (per serving):

- Calories: 220
- Protein: 20g
- Sodium: 300mg
- Potassium: 400mg
- Total Fat: 10g
- Saturated Fat: 2g
- Cholesterol: 120mg
- Carbohydrates: 10g
- Fiber: 3g
- Sugars: 3g

Egg Salad Lettuce Wraps

Prep Time: 15 minutes

Serving Size: 2 wraps

Ingredients:

- 4 large lettuce leaves (such as romaine or butter lettuce)
- 4 hard-boiled eggs, chopped
- 2 tbsp mayonnaise (choose a low-carb option)
- 1 tbsp Dijon mustard
- 2 tbsp chopped celery
- 2 tbsp chopped green onions
- Salt and pepper to taste

Instructions:

1. In a mixing bowl, combine the chopped hard-boiled eggs, mayonnaise, Dijon mustard, chopped celery, and chopped green onions.
2. Season with salt and pepper to taste and mix until well combined.
3. Lay out the lettuce leaves on a flat surface.
4. Divide the egg salad mixture evenly among the lettuce leaves.
5. Roll up each lettuce leaf into a wrap and serve immediately for a satisfying low-carb lunch.

Nutritional Information (per serving):

- Calories: 200
- Protein: 12g
- Sodium: 300mg
- Potassium: 200mg

- Total Fat: 15g

- Saturated Fat: 3g

- Cholesterol: 370mg

- Carbohydrates: 5g

- Fiber: 1g

- Sugars: 2g

Greek Salad with Grilled Chicken

Prep Time: 15 minutes

Cooking Time: 15 minutes

Serving Size: 1 salad

Ingredients:

- 4 oz grilled chicken breast, sliced

- 2 cups mixed greens (such as lettuce, spinach, and arugula)

- 1/4 cup cherry tomatoes, halved

- 1/4 cup cucumber, sliced

- 1/4 cup Kalamata olives, pitted

- 2 tbsp crumbled feta cheese

- 2 tbsp Greek dressing (look for a low-carb option)

- Salt and pepper to taste

Instructions:

1. Season the chicken breast with salt and pepper and grill until cooked through.

2. In a large bowl, combine the mixed greens, cherry tomatoes, cucumber, and Kalamata olives.

3. Add the sliced grilled chicken on top.

4. Sprinkle crumbled feta cheese over the salad.

5. Drizzle Greek dressing over the salad and toss to coat evenly.

6. Serve immediately as a flavorful and nutritious low-carb lunch option.

Nutritional Information (per serving):

- Calories: 280
- Protein: 30g
- Sodium: 500mg
- Potassium: 600mg
- Total Fat: 12g
- Saturated Fat: 3g
- Cholesterol: 80mg
- Carbohydrates: 10g
- Fiber: 3g
- Sugars: 4g

Salmon and Asparagus Foil Packets

Prep Time: 10 minutes

Cooking Time: 20 minutes

Serving Size: 1 packet

Ingredients:

- 4oz salmon fillet
- 8 spears asparagus, trimmed
- 1tbsp olive oil
- 1clove garlic, minced
- 1/2 tsp lemon zest

- Salt and pepper to taste

Instructions:

1. Preheat oven to 375°F.

2. Place each salmon fillet on a piece of aluminum foil large enough to fold over and seal.

3. Arrange asparagus spears next to the salmon fillets on the foil.

4. In a small bowl, whisk together olive oil, minced garlic, lemon zest, salt, and pepper.

5. Drizzle the olive oil mixture over the salmon and asparagus.

6. Fold the foil over the salmon and asparagus to create a packet and seal tightly.

7. Place the foil packets on a baking sheet and bake for 15-20 minutes until the salmon is cooked through and the asparagus is tender.

8. Carefully open the foil packets and serve immediately for a delicious and healthy low-carb lunch.

Nutritional Information (per serving):

- Calories: 280
- Protein: 25g
- Sodium: 300mg
- Potassium: 600mg
- Total Fat: 15g
- Saturated Fat: 3g
- Cholesterol: 80mg
- Carbohydrates: 5g
- Fiber: 2g

- Sugars: 2g

Caprese Stuffed Portobello Mushrooms

Prep Time: 15 minutes

Cooking Time: 20 minutes

Serving Size: 1 mushroom

Ingredients:

- 2 large portobello mushrooms
- 4 oz fresh mozzarella cheese, sliced
- 1/4 cup cherry tomatoes, halved
- 2 tbsp fresh basil leaves
- 1 tbsp balsamic glaze (look for a low-carb option)
- Salt and pepper to taste

Instructions:

1. Preheat oven to 375°F and line a baking sheet with parchment paper.
2. Remove the stems from the portobello mushrooms and gently scrape out the gills.
3. Place the mushrooms on the prepared baking sheet, gill side up.
4. Layer sliced mozzarella cheese, cherry tomatoes, and fresh basil leaves inside each mushroom.
5. Drizzle balsamic glaze over the stuffed mushrooms and season with salt and pepper to taste.
6. Bake for 15-20 minutes until the mushrooms are tender and the cheese is melted and bubbly.
7. Serve hot as a delicious and satisfying low-carb lunch option.

Nutritional Information (per serving):

- Calories: 250
- Protein: 20g
- Sodium: 400mg
- Potassium: 600mg
- Total Fat: 15g
- Saturated Fat: 6g
- Cholesterol: 30mg
- Carbohydrates: 8g
- Fiber: 2g
- Sugars: 4g

Cauliflower Fried Rice with Shrimp

Prep Time: 15 minutes

Cooking Time: 15 minutes

Serving Size: 1 serving

Ingredients:

- 1 cup cauliflower rice
- 6 large shrimp, peeled and deveined
- 1/4 cup diced carrots
- 1/4 cup diced bell peppers
- 1/4 cup diced onion
- 1 clove garlic, minced
- 1 egg, beaten
- 2 tbsp low-sodium soy sauce (or tamari for gluten-free)
- 1 tbsp sesame oil

- 1 green onion, chopped (for garnish)
- Salt and pepper to taste

Instructions:

1. Heat sesame oil in a large skillet or wok over medium heat.
2. Add minced garlic to the skillet and sauté until fragrant.
3. Add diced carrots, bell peppers, and onion to the skillet and stir-fry until tender.
4. Push the vegetables to one side of the skillet and pour the beaten egg into the empty space.
5. Scramble the egg until cooked through, then mix with the vegetables.
6. Add cauliflower rice and diced shrimp to the skillet.
7. Drizzle soy sauce over the mixture and toss to combine.
8. Cook for 5-7 minutes until the shrimp is cooked through and the cauliflower rice is tender.
9. Serve hot, garnished with chopped green onion, for a tasty low-carb lunch.

Nutritional Information (per serving):

- Calories: 220
- Protein: 20g
- Sodium: 500mg
- Potassium: 400mg
- Total Fat: 10g
- Saturated Fat: 2g
- Cholesterol: 180mg
- Carbohydrates: 10g

- Fiber: 3g
- Sugars: 4g

Turkey and Cheese Lettuce Wraps

Prep Time: 10 minutes

Serving Size: 2 wraps

Ingredients:

- 4 large lettuce leaves (such as romaine or butter lettuce)
- 6 oz sliced turkey breast
- 2 slices cheese (such as Swiss or cheddar)
- 1/4 cup sliced avocado
- 1/4 cup shredded carrots
- 1/4 cup sliced cucumber
- 2 tbsp ranch dressing (look for a low-carb option)
- Salt and pepper to taste

Instructions:

1. Lay out the lettuce leaves on a flat surface.
2. Place sliced turkey breast on each lettuce leaf.
3. Top with a slice of cheese, sliced avocado, shredded carrots, and sliced cucumber.
4. Drizzle ranch dressing over the toppings.
5. Season with salt and pepper to taste.
6. Roll up each lettuce leaf into a wrap and serve immediately for a quick and satisfying low-carb lunch.

Nutritional Information (per serving):

- Calories: 280

- Protein: 25g

- Sodium: 400mg

- Potassium: 600mg

- Total Fat: 15g

- Saturated Fat: 3g

- Cholesterol: 80mg

- Carbohydrates: 10g

- Fiber: 3g

- Sugars: 2g

Mediterranean Tuna Salad

Prep Time: 15 minutes

Serving Size: 1 salad

Ingredients:
- 1 can (5 oz) tuna in water, drained

- 2 cups mixed greens (such as lettuce, spinach, and arugula)

- 1/4 cup cherry tomatoes, halved

- 1/4 cup cucumber, sliced

- 2 tbsp Kalamata olives, pitted and halved

- 2 tbsp crumbled feta cheese

- 1 tbsp extra virgin olive oil

- 1 tbsp lemon juice

- 1/2 tsp dried oregano

- Salt and pepper to taste

Instructions:
1. In a large bowl, combine drained tuna, mixed greens, cherry tomatoes, cucumber, Kalamata olives, and crumbled feta cheese.

2. In a small bowl, whisk together extra virgin olive oil, lemon juice, dried oregano, salt, and pepper to make the dressing.

3. Drizzle the dressing over the salad and toss to coat evenly.

4. Serve immediately as a light and flavorful low-carb lunch option.

Nutritional Information (per serving):

- Calories: 250
- Protein: 25g
- Sodium: 500mg
- Potassium: 600mg
- Total Fat: 15g
- Saturated Fat: 3g
- Cholesterol: 40mg
- Carbohydrates: 8g
- Fiber: 3g
- Sugars: 3g

DINNER RECIPES

Grilled Salmon with Asparagus

Prep Time: 10 minutes

Cooking Time: 15 minutes

Serving Size: 1 fillet

Ingredients:

- 1 salmon fillet (6 oz)
- 1 tbsp olive oil
- 1/2 lemon, juiced
- 1 clove garlic, minced
- Salt and pepper to taste
- 1 cup asparagus spears, trimmed

Instructions:

1. Preheat grill to medium-high heat.
2. In a small bowl, whisk together olive oil, lemon juice, minced garlic, salt, and pepper.
3. Brush the salmon fillet and asparagus spears with the olive oil mixture.
4. Grill salmon for 5-7 minutes per side, or until cooked to desired doneness.
5. Grill asparagus for 3-4 minutes, turning occasionally, until tender.
6. Serve the grilled salmon alongside the asparagus for a flavorful low-carb dinner.

Nutritional Information (per serving):

- Calories: 300
- Protein: 30g
- Sodium: 200mg
- Potassium: 600mg
- Total Fat: 15g
- Saturated Fat: 2g
- Cholesterol: 80mg
- Carbohydrates: 5g
- Fiber: 2g
- Sugars: 2g

Cauliflower Fried Rice with Shrim

Prep Time: 15 minutes

Cooking Time: 10 minutes

Serving Size: 1 cup

Ingredients:

- 1/2 head cauliflower, grated
- 6 oz shrimp, peeled and deveined
- 1/4 cup diced carrots
- 1/4 cup diced bell peppers
- 1/4 cup diced onion
- 2 cloves garlic, minced
- 2 eggs, beaten
- 2 tbsp soy sauce (or tamari for gluten-free)
- 1 tbsp sesame oil

- 1 green onion, chopped (for garnish)
- Salt and pepper to taste

Instructions:

1. Heat sesame oil in a large skillet over medium heat.

2. Add diced onion, garlic, diced carrots, and diced bell peppers to the skillet. Cook for 2-3 minutes until softened.

3. Push the vegetables to one side of the skillet and add beaten eggs to the other side. Scramble the eggs until cooked through.

4. Stir in grated cauliflower and shrimp. Cook for 3-4 minutes until shrimp is pink and cauliflower is tender.

5. Pour soy sauce over the cauliflower mixture and toss to coat evenly.

6. Season with salt and pepper to taste.

7. Garnish with chopped green onions before serving.

Nutritional Information (per serving):
- Calories: 250
- Protein: 25g
- Sodium: 600mg
- Potassium: 400mg
- Total Fat: 10g
- Saturated Fat: 2g
- Cholesterol: 220mg
- Carbohydrates: 10g
- Fiber: 3g
- Sugars: 4g

Grilled Chicken Caesar Salad

Cooking Time: 15 minutes

Serving Size: 1 salad

Ingredients:

- 4 oz grilled chicken breast, sliced
- 2 cups romaine lettuce, chopped
- 1/4 cup cherry tomatoes, halved
- 2 tbsp grated Parmesan cheese
- 2 tbsp Caesar dressing (look for a low-carb option)
- 1 tbsp lemon juice
- 1/4 cup croutons (optional, use a low-carb alternative)
- Salt and pepper to taste

Instructions:

1. In a large bowl, combine chopped romaine lettuce, halved cherry tomatoes, and sliced grilled chicken breast.
2. Drizzle Caesar dressing and lemon juice over the salad.
3. Toss to coat evenly.
4. Sprinkle grated Parmesan cheese and croutons (if using) over the salad.
5. Season with salt and pepper to taste.
6. Serve immediately as a satisfying and low-carb dinner option.

Nutritional Information (per serving):

- Calories: 280
- Protein: 30g
- Sodium: 400mg

- Potassium: 400mg

- Total Fat: 12g

- Saturated Fat: 3g

- Cholesterol: 80mg

- Carbohydrates: 6g

- Fiber: 2g

- Sugars: 2g

Zucchini Lasagna

Prep Time: 20 minutes

Cooking Time: 45 minutes

Serving Size: 1 slice

Ingredients:

- 2 large zucchinis, sliced lengthwise into thin strips

- 1 lb ground beef or turkey

- 1 cup marinara sauce (look for a low-carb option)

- 1 cup ricotta cheese

- 1/2 cup grated Parmesan cheese

- 1 cup shredded mozzarella cheese

- 2 cloves garlic, minced

- 1 tsp dried oregano

- Salt and pepper to taste

Instructions:

1. Preheat oven to 375°F.

2. In a skillet, brown ground beef or turkey over medium heat. Drain excess fat.

3. Add minced garlic, dried oregano, salt, and pepper to the skillet. Stir until fragrant.

4. Stir in marinara sauce and simmer for 5 minutes.

5. In a separate bowl, mix together ricotta cheese and grated Parmesan cheese.

6. Spread a thin layer of marinara sauce on the bottom of a baking dish.

7. Layer zucchini strips over the sauce, followed by the meat sauce and ricotta mixture.

8. Repeat layers until all ingredients are used, finishing with a layer of zucchini strips on top.

9. Sprinkle shredded mozzarella cheese over the top layer.

10. Cover the baking dish with foil and bake for 30 minutes. Remove foil and bake for an additional 15 minutes until cheese is bubbly and golden.

11. Let the lasagna rest for 5-10 minutes before slicing and serving.

Nutritional Information (per serving):

- Calories: 350
- Protein: 30g
- Sodium: 500mg
- Potassium: 600mg
- Total Fat: 20g
- Saturated Fat: 10g
- Cholesterol: 90mg
- Carbohydrates: 10g

- Fiber: 3g

- Sugars: 5g

Turkey Stuffed Bell Peppers

Prep Time: 20 minutes

Cooking Time: 40 minutes

Serving Size: 1 stuffed pepper

Ingredients:

- 4 large bell peppers (any color), halved and seeded

- 1 lb ground turkey

- 1 cup cauliflower rice

- 1/2 cup diced tomatoes

- 1/4 cup diced onion

- 1/4 cup shredded mozzarella cheese

- 2 cloves garlic, minced

- 1 tsp Italian seasoning

- Salt and pepper to taste

Instructions:

1. Preheat oven to 375°F.

2. In a skillet, cook ground turkey over medium heat until browned. Drain excess fat.

3. Add minced garlic, diced onion, diced tomatoes, cauliflower rice, Italian seasoning, salt, and pepper to the skillet. Cook for 5-7 minutes until vegetables are tender.

4. Place bell pepper halves in a baking dish, cut side up.

5. Spoon turkey and vegetable mixture into each bell pepper half.

6. Sprinkle shredded mozzarella cheese over the stuffed peppers.

7. Cover the baking dish with foil and bake for 30 minutes.

8. Remove foil and bake for an additional 10 minutes until cheese is melted and bubbly.

9. Serve hot as a flavorful and low-carb dinner option.

Nutritional Information (per serving):

- Calories: 280
- Protein: 25g
- Sodium: 450mg
- Potassium: 600mg
- Total Fat: 15g
- Saturated Fat: 4g
- Cholesterol: 80mg
- Carbohydrates: 10g
- Fiber: 3g
- Sugars: 5g

Eggplant Parmesan

Prep Time: 30 minutes

Cooking Time: 45 minutes

Serving Size: 1 slice

Ingredients:

- 1 large eggplant, sliced into 1/2-inch rounds
- 2 eggs, beaten
- 1 cup almond flour
- 1 cup marinara sauce (look for a low-carb option)

- 1 cup shredded mozzarella cheese
- 1/2 cup grated Parmesan cheese
- 1/4 cup chopped fresh basil
- 2 cloves garlic, minced
- 1 tsp dried oregano
- Salt and pepper to taste

Instructions:

1. Preheat oven to 375°F. Line a baking sheet with parchment paper.
2. Dip eggplant slices in beaten eggs, then coat with almond flour. Place on the prepared baking sheet.
3. Bake eggplant slices for 15-20 minutes, flipping halfway through, until golden brown and tender.
4. In a mixing bowl, combine marinara sauce, minced garlic, dried oregano, salt, and pepper.
5. Spread a thin layer of marinara sauce on the bottom of a baking dish.
6. Arrange baked eggplant slices in the baking dish.
7. Top each eggplant slice with marinara sauce, shredded mozzarella cheese, and grated Parmesan cheese.
8. Bake for 20-25 minutes until cheese is melted and bubbly.
9. Garnish with chopped fresh basil before serving.

Nutritional Information (per serving):

- Calories: 320
- Protein: 20g
- Sodium: 600mg

- Potassium: 500mg
- Total Fat: 20g
- Saturated Fat: 6g
- Cholesterol: 100mg
- Carbohydrates: 10g
- Fiber: 5g
- Sugars: 4g

Spaghetti Squash with Pesto and Chicken

Prep Time: 10 minutes

Cooking Time: 40 minutes

Serving Size: 1 cup

Ingredients:

- 1 medium spaghetti squash, halved and seeded
- 1 lb boneless, skinless chicken breasts, cooked and shredded
- 1/2 cup basil pesto (look for a low-carb option)
- 1/4 cup grated Parmesan cheese
- 2 cloves garlic, minced
- 2 tbsp olive oil
- Salt and pepper to taste

Instructions:

1. Preheat oven to 400°F. Place spaghetti squash halves, cut side down, on a baking sheet lined with parchment paper.
2. Bake spaghetti squash for 30-40 minutes until tender. Use a fork to scrape the flesh into spaghetti-like strands.

3. In a skillet, heat olive oil over medium heat. Add minced garlic and cook until fragrant.

4. Add shredded chicken to the skillet and heat through.

5. Add cooked spaghetti squash strands to the skillet and toss to combine with the chicken.

6. Stir in basil pesto and grated Parmesan cheese. Cook for an additional 2-3 minutes until heated through.

7. Season with salt and pepper to taste.

8. Serve hot as a delicious and satisfying low-carb dinner option.

Nutritional Information (per serving):

- Calories: 320
- Protein: 25g
- Sodium: 400mg
- Potassium: 600mg
- Total Fat: 20g
- Saturated Fat: 4g
- Cholesterol: 80mg
- Carbohydrates: 10g
- Fiber: 3g
- Sugars: 4g

Stuffed Portobello Mushrooms

Prep Time: 15 minutes

Cooking Time: 25 minutes

Serving Size: 1 mushroom

Ingredients:

- 4 large portobello mushrooms, stems removed
- 1/2 lb Italian sausage, casing removed
- 1/2 cup marinara sauce (look for a low-carb option)
- 1/2 cup shredded mozzarella cheese
- 1/4 cup grated Parmesan cheese
- 1/4 cup chopped fresh parsley
- 2 cloves garlic, minced
- 1 tbsp olive oil
- Salt and pepper to taste

Instructions:

1. Preheat oven to 375°F. Line a baking sheet with parchment paper.
2. Place portobello mushrooms on the prepared baking sheet, gill side up.
3. In a skillet, heat olive oil over medium heat. Add minced garlic and cook until fragrant.
4. Add Italian sausage to the skillet and cook until browned and cooked through. Drain excess fat.
5. Stir in marinara sauce and chopped fresh parsley. Cook for 2-3 minutes until heated through.
6. Spoon the sausage mixture into each portobello mushroom cap.
7. Sprinkle shredded mozzarella cheese and grated Parmesan cheese over the stuffed mushrooms.

8. Bake for 20-25 minutes until cheese is melted and mushrooms are tender.

9. Serve hot as a flavorful and low-carb dinner option.

Nutritional Information (per serving):

- Calories: 300
- Protein: 20g
- Sodium: 600mg
- Potassium: 800mg
- Total Fat: 20g
- Saturated Fat: 8g
- Cholesterol: 60mg
- Carbohydrates: 10g
- Fiber: 3g
- Sugars: 4g

Lemon Garlic Butter Shrimp with Zoodles

Prep Time: 15 minutes

Cooking Time: 10 minutes

Serving Size: 1 cup

Ingredients:

- 1 lb large shrimp, peeled and deveined
- 4 medium zucchinis, spiralized into noodles (zoodles)
- 4 tbsp unsalted butter
- 4 cloves garlic, minced
- 1/4 cup chicken broth
- 1/4 cup chopped fresh parsley

- 1 lemon, juiced and zest
- Salt and pepper to taste

Instructions:

1. In a large skillet, melt butter over medium heat. Add minced garlic and cook until fragrant.
2. Add shrimp to the skillet and cook for 2-3 minutes per side until pink and opaque.
3. Remove shrimp from the skillet and set aside.
4. In the same skillet, add chicken broth, lemon juice, and lemon zest. Bring to a simmer.
5. Add spiralized zucchini noodles (zoodles) to the skillet and toss to coat in the lemon garlic butter sauce. Cook for 2-3 minutes until zoodles are tender.
6. Return cooked shrimp to the skillet and toss to combine with the zoodles.
7. Season with salt and pepper to taste.
8. Garnish with chopped fresh parsley before serving.

Nutritional Information (per serving):

- Calories: 250
- Protein: 25g
- Sodium: 500mg
- Potassium: 800mg
- Total Fat: 12g
- Saturated Fat: 6g
- Cholesterol: 200mg
- Carbohydrates: 10g

- Fiber: 3g

- Sugars: 4g

Greek Salad with Grilled Chicken

Prep Time: 15 minutes

Cooking Time: 15 minutes

Serving Size: 1 salad

Ingredients:

- 4 oz grilled chicken breast, sliced

- 2 cups mixed greens (romaine, spinach, arugula, etc.)

- 1/4 cup cucumber, sliced

- 1/4 cup cherry tomatoes, halved

- 1/4 cup Kalamata olives

- 1/4 cup crumbled feta cheese

- 2 tbsp extra virgin olive oil

- 1 tbsp red wine vinegar

- 1/2 tsp dried oregano

- Salt and pepper to taste

Instructions:

1. In a large bowl, combine mixed greens, sliced cucumber, halved cherry tomatoes, Kalamata olives, and crumbled feta cheese.

2. Drizzle extra virgin olive oil and red wine vinegar over the salad.

3. Sprinkle dried oregano, salt, and pepper over the salad.

4. Toss to coat evenly.

5. Top the salad with sliced grilled chicken breast.

6. Serve immediately as a refreshing and low-carb dinner option.

Nutritional Information (per serving):

- Calories: 280
- Protein: 25g
- Sodium: 600mg
- Potassium: 400mg
- Total Fat: 15g
- Saturated Fat: 4g
- Cholesterol: 80mg
- Carbohydrates: 10g
- Fiber: 3g
- Sugars: 4g

SNACK RECIPES

Cucumber and Cream Cheese Roll-Ups

Prep Time: 10 minutes

Serving Size: 4 roll-ups

Ingredients:

- 1 large cucumber
- 4 tbsp cream cheese
- 4 slices smoked salmon or deli turkey
- 1 tbsp chopped fresh dill (optional)
- Salt and pepper to taste

Instructions:

1. Wash the cucumber and slice it lengthwise into thin strips using a mandoline or vegetable peeler.
2. Pat the cucumber strips dry with a paper towel to remove excess moisture.
3. Spread 1 tablespoon of cream cheese evenly onto each cucumber strip.
4. Place a slice of smoked salmon or deli turkey on top of the cream cheese.
5. Sprinkle chopped fresh dill over the salmon or turkey, if desired.
6. Season with salt and pepper to taste.
7. Roll up each cucumber strip tightly, starting from one end.
8. Secure the roll-ups with toothpicks if necessary.
9. Serve immediately or refrigerate until ready to serve.

Nutritional Information (per serving):

- Calories: 70
- Protein: 4g
- Sodium: 180mg
- Potassium: 200mg
- Total Fat: 5g
- Saturated Fat: 2.5g
- Cholesterol: 15mg
- Carbohydrates: 2g
- Fiber: 0g
- Sugars: 1g

Avocado and Tuna Stuffed Mini Bell Peppers

Prep Time: 15 minutes

Serving Size: 2 stuffed peppers

Ingredients:

- 4 mini bell peppers
- 1 avocado, mashed
- 1 can (5 oz) tuna, drained
- 1 tbsp Greek yogurt or mayonnaise
- 1 tbsp lemon juice
- 1/4 tsp garlic powder
- Salt and pepper to taste
- Chopped fresh parsley for garnish (optional)

Instructions:

1. Cut the mini bell peppers in half lengthwise and remove the seeds and membranes.

2. In a bowl, mix together mashed avocado, drained tuna, Greek yogurt or mayonnaise, lemon juice, garlic powder, salt, and pepper.

3. Spoon the avocado and tuna mixture into each bell pepper half.

4. Garnish with chopped fresh parsley, if desired.

5. Serve immediately or refrigerate until ready to serve.

Nutritional Information (per serving):

- Calories: 160
- Protein: 14g
- Sodium: 180mg
- Potassium: 470mg
- Total Fat: 8g
- Saturated Fat: 1.5g
- Cholesterol: 15mg
- Carbohydrates: 9g
- Fiber: 5g
- Sugars: 3g

Cheese and Veggie Skewers

Prep Time: 10 minutes

Serving Size: 2 skewers

Ingredients:

- 4 cherry tomatoes
- 4 cubes of cheese (such as cheddar, mozzarella, or Swiss)
- 4 cucumber slices
- 4 black olives
- 4 slices of salami or pepperoni (optional)
- 2 wooden skewers

Instructions:

1. Thread cherry tomatoes, cheese cubes, cucumber slices, black olives, and salami or pepperoni (if using) onto the wooden skewers in any desired order.
2. Repeat until all ingredients are used, making 2 skewers in total.
3. Serve immediately or refrigerate until ready to serve.

Nutritional Information (per serving):

- Calories: 120
- Protein: 6g
- Sodium: 250mg
- Potassium: 180mg
- Total Fat: 8g
- Saturated Fat: 4g
- Cholesterol: 20mg
- Carbohydrates: 4g
- Fiber: 1g
- Sugars: 2g

Almond Butter and Celery Sticks

Prep Time: 5 minutes

Serving Size: 2 celery sticks

Ingredients:

- 2 celery stalks
- 2 tbsp almond butter
- 1 tbsp unsweetened shredded coconut (optional)
- 1 tbsp sliced almonds (optional)
- 1/2 tsp ground cinnamon (optional)

Instructions:

1. Wash the celery stalks and cut them into halves or thirds, depending on their length.
2. Spread almond butter onto each celery stick.
3. Sprinkle unsweetened shredded coconut, sliced almonds, and ground cinnamon on top of the almond butter, if desired.
4. Serve immediately.

   Nutritional Information (per serving):

- Calories: 120
- Protein: 3g
- Sodium: 65mg
- Potassium: 260mg
- Total Fat: 10g
- Saturated Fat: 1g
- Cholesterol: 0mg
- Carbohydrates: 5g

- Fiber: 3g
- Sugars: 2g

Greek Yogurt and Berry Parfait

Prep Time: 5 minutes

Serving Size: 1 parfait

Ingredients:

- 1/2 cup Greek yogurt
- 1/4 cup mixed berries (such as strawberries, blueberries, raspberries)
- 1 tbsp unsweetened granola
- 1 tsp honey (optional)

Instructions:

1. In a serving glass or bowl, layer half of the Greek yogurt.
2. Add half of the mixed berries on top of the yogurt layer.
3. Sprinkle half of the unsweetened granola over the berries.
4. Repeat the layers with the remaining Greek yogurt, mixed berries, and granola.
5. Drizzle honey on top for extra sweetness, if desired.
6. Serve immediately.

Nutritional Information (per serving):

- Calories: 160
- Protein: 14g
- Sodium: 60mg
- Potassium: 170mg
- Total Fat: 4g

- Saturated Fat: 0g
- Cholesterol: 10mg
- Carbohydrates: 20g
- Fiber: 3g
- Sugars: 14g

CHAPTER 4

MODERATE CARB DAYS: RECIPES

BREAKFAST RECIPES

Spinach and Feta Breakfast Wrap

Prep Time: 10 minutes

Cooking Time: 10 minutes

Serving Size: 1 wrap

Ingredients:

- 1 whole wheat tortilla
- 2 eggs
- 1/4 cup spinach, chopped
- 2 tbsp feta cheese, crumbled
- Salt and pepper to taste
- Cooking spray

Instructions:

1. In a bowl, whisk together eggs, spinach, feta cheese, salt, and pepper.
2. Heat a non-stick skillet over medium heat and coat with cooking spray.
3. Pour the egg mixture into the skillet and cook until the eggs are set, stirring occasionally.
4. Warm the tortilla in a separate skillet or microwave.

5. Once the eggs are cooked, place them onto the warmed tortilla.

6. Roll up the tortilla, folding in the sides to create a wrap.

7. Serve immediately.

Nutritional Information (per serving):

- Calories: 280
- Protein: 18g
- Sodium: 590mg
- Potassium: 230mg
- Total Fat: 14g
- Saturated Fat: 5g
- Cholesterol: 390mg
- Carbohydrates: 19g
- Fiber: 3g
- Sugars: 1g

Mediterranean Avocado Toast

Prep Time: 5 minutes

Cooking Time: 5 minutes

Serving Size: 1 toast

Ingredients:

- 1 slice whole grain bread
- 1/2 avocado, mashed
- 2 slices tomato
- 1 tbsp feta cheese, crumbled
- 1 tsp olive oil
- Salt and pepper to taste

Instructions:

1. Toast the slice of whole grain bread until golden brown.
2. Spread the mashed avocado evenly on the toast.
3. Top with slices of tomato and crumbled feta cheese.
4. Drizzle with olive oil and season with salt and pepper.
5. Serve immediately.

Nutritional Information (per serving):

- Calories: 230
- Protein: 7g
- Sodium: 290mg
- Potassium: 490mg
- Total Fat: 15g
- Saturated Fat: 3g
- Cholesterol: 5mg
- Carbohydrates: 20g
- Fiber: 6g
- Sugars: 2g

Greek Yogurt Parfait

Prep Time: 5 minutes

Serving Size: 1 parfait

Ingredients:

- 1/2 cup Greek yogurt
- 1/4 cup granola
- 1/4 cup mixed berries (strawberries, blueberries, raspberries)
- 1 tbsp honey

Instructions:

1. In a glass, layer Greek yogurt, granola, and mixed berries.
2. Drizzle honey over the top.
3. Repeat the layers if desired.
4. Serve immediately.

Nutritional Information (per serving):

- Calories: 280
- Protein: 15g
- Sodium: 60mg
- Potassium: 290mg
- Total Fat: 6g
- Saturated Fat: 1g
- Cholesterol: 5mg
- Carbohydrates: 45g
- Fiber: 6g
- Sugars: 20g

Quinoa Breakfast Bowl

Prep Time: 5 minutes

Cooking Time: 15 minutes

Serving Size: 1 bowl

Ingredients:

- 1/2 cup cooked quinoa
- 1/4 cup unsweetened almond milk
- 1/4 cup sliced strawberries
- 1/4 cup sliced banana
- 1 tbsp almond butter
- 1 tsp honey
- Pinch of cinnamon

Instructions:

1. In a small saucepan, heat the cooked quinoa with almond milk until warm.
2. Transfer the quinoa to a bowl.
3. Top with sliced strawberries, banana, almond butter, honey, and a pinch of cinnamon.
4. Serve warm.

Nutritional Information (per serving):

- Calories: 320
- Protein: 8g
- Sodium: 60mg
- Potassium: 450mg
- Total Fat: 9g
- Saturated Fat: 1g

- Cholesterol: 0mg

- Carbohydrates: 55g

- Fiber: 6g

- Sugars: 16g

Sweet Potato Hash

Prep Time: 10 minutes

Cooking Time: 20 minutes

Serving Size: 1 cup

Ingredients:

- 1 medium sweet potato, peeled and diced

- 1/4 cup onion, diced

- 1/4 cup bell pepper, diced

- 2 slices turkey bacon, diced

- 1 tsp olive oil

- Salt and pepper to taste

- 1/4 tsp paprika (optional)

Instructions:

1. Heat olive oil in a skillet over medium heat.

2. Add diced sweet potato and cook until slightly softened, about 5 minutes.

3. Add diced onion, bell pepper, and turkey bacon to the skillet.

4. Season with salt, pepper, and paprika if desired.

5. Cook, stirring occasionally, until sweet potatoes are tender and bacon is crispy, about 10-15 minutes.

6. Serve hot.

Nutritional Information (per serving):

- Calories: 240
- Protein: 8g
- Sodium: 350mg
- Potassium: 560mg
- Total Fat: 7g
- Saturated Fat: 1.5g
- Cholesterol: 15mg
- Carbohydrates: 35g
- Fiber: 6g
- Sugars: 8g

Cottage Cheese Pancakes

Prep Time: 10 minutes

Cooking Time: 10 minutes

Serving Size: 2 pancakes

Ingredients:

- 1/2 cup cottage cheese
- 2 eggs
- 1/4 cup oat flour
- 1/2 tsp vanilla extract
- Cooking spray

Instructions:

1. In a blender, combine cottage cheese, eggs, oat flour, and vanilla extract. Blend until smooth.

2. Heat a non-stick skillet over medium heat and coat with cooking spray.

3. Pour small circles of batter onto the skillet to form pancakes.

4. Cook until bubbles form on the surface, then flip and cook until golden brown on both sides.

5. Repeat with the remaining batter.

6. Serve hot with your choice of toppings.

Nutritional Information (per serving):

- Calories: 260
- Protein: 23g
- Sodium: 380mg
- Potassium: 200mg
- Total Fat: 11g
- Saturated Fat: 4g
- Cholesterol: 390mg
- Carbohydrates: 17g
- Fiber: 2g
- Sugars: 3g

Veggie Omelette

Prep Time: 10 minutes

Cooking Time: 10 minutes

Serving Size: 1 omelette

Ingredients:

- 2 eggs
- 1/4 cup diced bell peppers (any color)

- 1/4 cup diced onions
- 1/4 cup diced tomatoes
- 1/4 cup diced mushrooms
- 1/4 cup shredded cheddar cheese
- Salt and pepper to taste
- Cooking spray

Instructions:

1. In a bowl, beat the eggs until well mixed.
2. Heat a non-stick skillet over medium heat and coat with cooking spray.
3. Pour the beaten eggs into the skillet.
4. As the eggs begin to set, add the diced vegetables evenly over the surface of the omelette.
5. Sprinkle shredded cheese over the vegetables.
6. When the edges of the omelette start to lift from the skillet, fold it in half using a spatula.
7. Cook for another minute or until the cheese is melted and the omelette is cooked through.
8. Slide the omelette onto a plate and serve hot.

Nutritional Information (per serving):

- Calories: 280
- Protein: 20g
- Sodium: 370mg
- Potassium: 430mg
- Total Fat: 17g
- Saturated Fat: 7g

- Cholesterol: 390mg

- Carbohydrates: 11g

- Fiber: 3g

- Sugars: 5g

Protein-Packed Breakfast Burrito

Prep Time: 10 minutes

Cooking Time: 10 minutes

Serving Size: 1 burrito

Ingredients:

- 1 whole wheat tortilla

- 2 eggs, scrambled

- 1/4 cup black beans, drained and rinsed

- 1/4 cup diced tomatoes

- 1/4 cup diced avocado

- 2 tbsp salsa

- Salt and pepper to taste

Instructions:

1. Heat the whole wheat tortilla in a skillet or microwave until warm.

2. Place scrambled eggs, black beans, diced tomatoes, and diced avocado in the center of the tortilla.

3. Drizzle salsa over the filling.

4. Season with salt and pepper to taste.

5. Fold in the sides of the tortilla and roll it up into a burrito.

6. Serve immediately.

Nutritional Information (per serving):

- Calories: 340
- Protein: 20g
- Sodium: 550mg
- Potassium: 590mg
- Total Fat: 15g
- Saturated Fat: 3.5g
- Cholesterol: 390mg
- Carbohydrates: 35g
- Fiber: 9g
- Sugars: 3g

Chia Seed Pudding

Prep Time: 5 minutes (plus chilling time)

Serving Size: 1 pudding cup

Ingredients:

- 2 tbsp chia seeds
- 1/2 cup unsweetened almond milk
- 1/2 tsp vanilla extract
- 1 tsp honey or maple syrup (optional)
- Fresh fruit for topping (such as berries or sliced banana)
- Nuts or seeds for topping (such as almonds or pumpkin seeds)

Instructions:

- In a small bowl or jar, combine chia seeds, almond milk, vanilla extract, and honey or maple syrup if using.

- Stir well to combine.
- Cover the bowl or jar and refrigerate for at least 2 hours or overnight, until the chia seeds have absorbed the liquid and the mixture has thickened to a pudding-like consistency.
- Once chilled, give the pudding a stir to redistribute the chia seeds.
- Transfer the pudding to a serving cup or bowl.
- Top with fresh fruit and nuts or seeds as desired.
- Serve chilled.

Nutritional Information (per serving):

- Calories: 170
- Protein: 5g
- Sodium: 80mg
- Potassium: 120mg
- Total Fat: 9g
- Saturated Fat: 1g
- Cholesterol: 0mg
- Carbohydrates: 17g
- Fiber: 8g
- Sugars: 6g

Breakfast Egg Muffins

Prep Time: 10 minutes

Cooking Time: 20 minutes

Serving Size: 2 muffins

Ingredients:

- 4 eggs
- 1/4 cup diced bell peppers (any color)
- 1/4 cup diced onions
- 1/4 cup diced tomatoes
- 1/4 cup chopped spinach
- 1/4 cup shredded cheddar cheese
- Salt and pepper to taste
- Cooking spray

Instructions:

- Preheat the oven to 350°F (175°C). Grease a muffin tin with cooking spray.
- In a bowl, whisk together the eggs until well beaten.
- Stir in the diced bell peppers, onions, tomatoes, spinach, and shredded cheddar cheese. Season with salt and pepper to taste.
- Divide the egg mixture evenly among the muffin cups.
- Bake in the preheated oven for 15-20 minutes, or until the egg muffins are set and lightly golden on top.
- Remove from the oven and let cool for a few minutes before serving.
- Serve warm or at room temperature.

Nutritional Information (per serving, 2 muffins):

- Calories: 220
- Protein: 15g
- Sodium: 290mg

- Potassium: 310mg

- Total Fat: 14g

- Saturated Fat: 6g

- Cholesterol: 385mg

- Carbohydrates: 8g

- Fiber: 2g

- Sugars: 4g

LUNCH RECIPES

Turkey and Avocado Wrap

Prep Time: 10 minutes

Serving Size: 1 wrap

Ingredients:

- 1 whole wheat tortilla
- 3 oz sliced turkey breast
- 1/4 avocado, sliced
- 1/4 cup shredded lettuce
- 2 slices tomato
- 1 tbsp hummus
- Salt and pepper to taste

Instructions:

1. Lay the whole wheat tortilla flat on a clean surface.
2. Spread hummus evenly over the tortilla.
3. Layer sliced turkey breast, avocado, shredded lettuce, and tomato slices on top of the hummus.
4. Season with salt and pepper to taste.
5. Roll up the tortilla tightly, folding in the sides to create a wrap.
6. Slice in half diagonally, if desired, and serve immediately.

Nutritional Information (per serving):

- Calories: 320
- Protein: 25g
- Sodium: 540mg

- Potassium: 370mg

- Total Fat: 12g

- Saturated Fat: 2g

- Cholesterol: 35mg

- Carbohydrates: 30g

- Fiber: 8g

- Sugars: 3g

Mediterranean Quinoa Salad

Prep Time: 15 minutes

Cooking Time: 15 minutes

Serving Size: 1 bowl

Ingredients:

- 1/2 cup quinoa, uncooked

- 1 cup water

- 1/4 cup diced cucumber

- 1/4 cup diced tomatoes

- 1/4 cup diced bell peppers (any color)

- 2 tbsp chopped fresh parsley

- 2 tbsp crumbled feta cheese

- 1 tbsp extra virgin olive oil

- 1 tbsp lemon juice

- Salt and pepper to taste

Instructions:

1. Rinse the quinoa under cold water. In a saucepan, combine
   quinoa and water. Bring to a boil, then reduce heat to low,

cover, and simmer for 15 minutes, or until quinoa is cooked and water is absorbed.

2. Fluff the cooked quinoa with a fork and let it cool slightly.

3. In a large bowl, combine the cooked quinoa, diced cucumber, tomatoes, bell peppers, parsley, and crumbled feta cheese.

4. Drizzle with olive oil and lemon juice. Season with salt and pepper to taste.

5. Toss well to combine.

6. Serve at room temperature or chilled.

Nutritional Information (per serving):

- Calories: 280
- Protein: 9g
- Sodium: 190mg
- Potassium: 330mg
- Total Fat: 10g
- Saturated Fat: 2g
- Cholesterol: 5mg
- Carbohydrates: 38g
- Fiber: 5g
- Sugars: 2g

Grilled Chicken Caesar Salad

Prep Time: 15 minutes

Cooking Time: 15 minutes

Serving Size: 1 salad

Ingredients:

- 4 oz grilled chicken breast, sliced
- 2 cups chopped romaine lettuce
- 1/4 cup cherry tomatoes, halved
- 2 tbsp grated Parmesan cheese
- 2 tbsp Caesar dressing
- 1/4 cup croutons

Instructions:

1. Season the chicken breast with salt and pepper, then grill until cooked through, about 6-7 minutes per side. Let it rest for a few minutes, then slice.
2. In a large bowl, combine the chopped romaine lettuce, cherry tomatoes, and sliced grilled chicken.
3. Drizzle with Caesar dressing and toss to coat evenly.
4. Sprinkle grated Parmesan cheese and croutons over the salad.
5. Serve immediately.

Nutritional Information (per serving):

- Calories: 340
- Protein: 30g
- Sodium: 590mg
- Potassium: 550mg
- Total Fat: 15g
- Saturated Fat: 3g
- Cholesterol: 80mg
- Carbohydrates: 20g

- Fiber: 4g
- Sugars: 3g

Veggie and Hummus Wrap

Prep Time: 10 minutes

Serving Size: 1 wrap

Ingredients:

- 1 whole wheat tortilla
- 2 tbsp hummus
- 1/4 cup shredded lettuce
- 1/4 cup sliced cucumber
- 1/4 cup shredded carrots
- 2 slices tomato
- 2 slices red onion
- Salt and pepper to taste

Instructions:

1. Spread hummus evenly over the whole wheat tortilla.
2. Layer shredded lettuce, sliced cucumber, shredded carrots, tomato slices, and red onion slices on top of the hummus.
3. Season with salt and pepper to taste.
4. Roll up the tortilla tightly, folding in the sides to create a wrap.
5. Slice in half diagonally, if desired, and serve immediately.

Nutritional Information (per serving):

- Calories: 240
- Protein: 7g
- Sodium: 430mg

- Potassium: 370mg

- Total Fat: 7g

- Saturated Fat: 1g

- Cholesterol: 0mg

- Carbohydrates: 38g

- Fiber: 8g

- Sugars: 5g

Lentil and Vegetable Soup

Prep Time: 15 minutes

Cooking Time: 30 minutes

Serving Size: 1 bowl

Ingredients:

- 1/2 cup dried green lentils

- 4 cups vegetable broth

- 1/2 cup diced onion

- 1/2 cup diced carrots

- 1/2 cup diced celery

- 1/2 cup diced bell peppers (any color)

- 2 cloves garlic, minced

- 1 tsp olive oil

- 1/2 tsp dried thyme

- 1/2 tsp dried oregano

- Salt and pepper to taste

- Fresh parsley for garnish (optional)

Instructions:

1. Rinse the dried green lentils under cold water and drain.

2. In a large pot, heat olive oil over medium heat. Add diced onion, carrots, celery, bell peppers, and garlic. Cook until vegetables are softened, about 5-7 minutes.

3. Add dried lentils, vegetable broth, dried thyme, and dried oregano to the pot. Bring to a boil, then reduce heat to low, cover, and simmer for 25-30 minutes, or until lentils are tender.

4. Season with salt and pepper to taste.

5. Ladle the soup into serving bowls and garnish with fresh parsley if desired.

6. Serve hot.

Nutritional Information (per serving):

- Calories: 220
- Protein: 14g
- Sodium: 680mg
- Potassium: 520mg
- Total Fat: 3g
- Saturated Fat: 0g
- Cholesterol: 0mg
- Carbohydrates: 36g
- Fiber: 15g
- Sugars: 6g

Chickpea Salad Sandwich

Prep Time: 10 minutes

Serving Size: 1 sandwich

Ingredients:

- 1/2 cup canned chickpeas, drained and rinsed
- 1 tbsp Greek yogurt
- 1 tbsp diced red onion
- 1 tbsp diced celery
- 1 tbsp chopped fresh parsley
- 1/2 tsp Dijon mustard
- Salt and pepper to taste
- 2 slices whole grain bread
- Lettuce leaves and tomato slices for serving

Instructions:

1. In a bowl, mash the chickpeas with a fork until slightly chunky.
2. Add Greek yogurt, diced red onion, diced celery, chopped parsley, Dijon mustard, salt, and pepper to the mashed chickpeas. Mix well to combine.
3. Toast the slices of whole grain bread, if desired.
4. Spread the chickpea salad mixture evenly onto one slice of bread.
5. Top with lettuce leaves and tomato slices, then cover with the other slice of bread.
6. Slice the sandwich in half, if desired, and serve immediately.

Nutritional Information (per serving):

- Calories: 280

- Protein: 12g

- Sodium: 440mg

- Potassium: 360mg

- Total Fat: 4g

- Saturated Fat: 0.5g

- Cholesterol: 0mg

- Carbohydrates: 51g

- Fiber: 10g

- Sugars: 7g

Caprese Quinoa Bowl

Prep Time: 15 minutes

Cooking Time: 15 minutes

Serving Size: 1 bowl

Ingredients:

- 1/2 cup quinoa, uncooked

- 1 cup water

- 1/2 cup cherry tomatoes, halved

- 1/4 cup fresh mozzarella balls, halved

- 2 tbsp chopped fresh basil

- 1 tbsp balsamic glaze

- Salt and pepper to taste

Instructions:

1. Rinse the quinoa under cold water. In a saucepan, combine quinoa and water. Bring to a boil, then reduce heat to low,

cover, and simmer for 15 minutes, or until quinoa is cooked and water is absorbed.

2. Fluff the cooked quinoa with a fork and let it cool slightly.

3. In a bowl, combine the cooked quinoa, cherry tomatoes, fresh mozzarella balls, and chopped basil.

4. Drizzle with balsamic glaze. Season with salt and pepper to taste.

5. Toss well to combine.

6. Serve at room temperature or chilled.

Nutritional Information (per serving):

- Calories: 320
- Protein: 12g
- Sodium: 120mg
- Potassium: 400mg
- Total Fat: 10g
- Saturated Fat: 4g
- Cholesterol: 20mg
- Carbohydrates: 45g
- Fiber: 5g
- Sugars: 4g

Veggie Stir-Fry with Tofu

Prep Time: 15 minutes

Cooking Time: 15 minutes

Serving Size: 1 plate

Ingredients:

- 1/2 cup firm tofu, cubed
- 1 cup mixed vegetables (bell peppers, broccoli, carrots, snap peas)
- 1 clove garlic, minced
- 1 tbsp soy sauce
- 1 tsp sesame oil
- 1/2 tsp grated ginger
- Cooked brown rice for serving

Instructions:

1. Heat sesame oil in a large skillet or wok over medium-high heat.
2. Add minced garlic and grated ginger to the skillet. Cook for 1 minute, until fragrant.
3. Add cubed tofu to the skillet. Stir-fry for 5-6 minutes, until tofu is golden brown and crispy.
4. Add mixed vegetables to the skillet. Stir-fry for 4-5 minutes, until vegetables are tender-crisp.
5. Pour soy sauce over the tofu and vegetables. Stir well to combine.
6. Serve the stir-fry hot over cooked brown rice.

Nutritional Information (per serving):

- Calories: 320
- Protein: 18g
- Sodium: 580mg
- Potassium: 520mg

- Total Fat: 12g

- Saturated Fat: 2g

- Cholesterol: 0mg

- Carbohydrates: 38g

- Fiber: 6g

- Sugars: 4g

Mediterranean Pasta Salad

Prep Time: 15 minutes

Cooking Time: 10 minutes

Serving Size: 1 bowl

Ingredients:

- 1/2 cup whole wheat pasta, uncooked

- 1/4 cup diced cucumber

- 1/4 cup halved cherry tomatoes

- 2 tbsp diced red onion

- 2 tbsp sliced Kalamata olives

- 1 tbsp crumbled feta cheese

- 1 tbsp extra virgin olive oil

- 1 tbsp lemon juice

- 1/2 tsp dried oregano

- Salt and pepper to taste

Instructions:

1. Cook the whole wheat pasta according to package instructions. Drain and let it cool slightly.

2. In a large bowl, combine the cooked pasta, diced cucumber, cherry tomatoes, red onion, sliced Kalamata olives, and crumbled feta cheese.

3. Drizzle with extra virgin olive oil and lemon juice. Sprinkle dried oregano over the salad.

4. Season with salt and pepper to taste.

5. Toss well to combine.

6. Serve at room temperature or chilled.

Nutritional Information (per serving):

- Calories: 280

- Protein: 8g

- Sodium: 230mg

- Potassium: 220mg

- Total Fat: 9g

- Saturated Fat: 2g

- Cholesterol: 5mg

- Carbohydrates: 40g

- Fiber: 6g

- Sugars: 3g

Asian-style Tofu and Vegetable Stir-Fry

Prep Time: 15 minutes

Cooking Time: 15 minutes

Serving Size: 1 plate

Ingredients:

- 1/2 cup firm tofu, cubed

- 1 cup mixed vegetables (bell peppers, broccoli, carrots, snap peas)
- 2 cloves garlic, minced
- 1 tbsp soy sauce
- 1 tbsp hoisin sauce
- 1/2 tsp sesame oil
- Cooked brown rice for serving

Instructions:

1. Heat sesame oil in a large skillet or wok over medium-high heat.
2. Add minced garlic to the skillet. Cook for 1 minute, until fragrant.
3. Add cubed tofu to the skillet. Stir-fry for 5-6 minutes, until tofu is golden brown and crispy.
4. Add mixed vegetables to the skillet. Stir-fry for 4-5 minutes, until vegetables are tender-crisp.
5. In a small bowl, mix together soy sauce and hoisin sauce. Pour the sauce mixture over the tofu and vegetables in the skillet.
6. Stir well to combine and coat evenly.
7. Serve the stir-fry hot over cooked brown rice.

Nutritional Information (per serving):

- Calories: 320
- Protein: 18g
- Sodium: 680mg
- Potassium: 520mg

- Total Fat: 12g
- Saturated Fat: 2g
- Cholesterol: 0mg
- Carbohydrates: 38g
- Fiber: 6g
- Sugars: 5g

DINNER RECIPES

Lemon Herb Grilled Salmon

Prep Time: 10 minutes

Cooking Time: 10 minutes

Serving Size: 1 fillet

Ingredients:

- 1 salmon fillet (6 oz)
- 1 tbsp olive oil
- 1 tbsp lemon juice
- 1 clove garlic, minced
- 1/2 tsp dried thyme
- 1/2 tsp dried rosemary
- Salt and pepper to taste
- Lemon slices for garnish

Instructions:

1. In a small bowl, whisk together olive oil, lemon juice, minced garlic, dried thyme, and dried rosemary.
2. Season the salmon fillet with salt and pepper on both sides.
3. Place the salmon fillet in a shallow dish and pour the marinade over it. Allow it to marinate for 15-30 minutes in the refrigerator.
4. Preheat the grill to medium-high heat.
5. Remove the salmon from the marinade and discard any excess marinade.

6. Place the salmon fillet on the preheated grill and cook for 4-5 minutes per side, or until the fish flakes easily with a fork.

7. Transfer the grilled salmon to a serving plate, garnish with lemon slices, and serve hot.

Nutritional Information (per serving):

- Calories: 320
- Protein: 34g
- Sodium: 110mg
- Potassium: 850mg
- Total Fat: 18g
- Saturated Fat: 3g
- Cholesterol: 95mg
- Carbohydrates: 2g
- Fiber: 0g
- Sugars: 0g

Quinoa Stuffed Bell Peppers

Prep Time: 15 minutes

Cooking Time: 30 minutes

Serving Size: 1 stuffed pepper

Ingredients:

- 2 large bell peppers (any color)
- 1/2 cup quinoa, uncooked
- 1 cup water or vegetable broth
- 1/2 cup black beans, drained and rinsed
- 1/2 cup corn kernels (fresh, canned, or frozen)

- 1/4 cup diced tomatoes
- 1/4 cup diced red onion
- 1/4 cup shredded cheddar cheese
- 1 tsp olive oil
- 1/2 tsp ground cumin
- Salt and pepper to taste

Instructions:

1. Preheat oven to 375°F (190°C).
2. Cut the tops off the bell peppers and remove the seeds and membranes.
3. In a saucepan, bring water or vegetable broth to a boil. Add quinoa, cover, and simmer for 15-20 minutes until quinoa is cooked and liquid is absorbed.
4. In a skillet, heat olive oil over medium heat. Add diced red onion and cook until softened, about 3-4 minutes.
5. Add cooked quinoa, black beans, corn kernels, diced tomatoes, shredded cheddar cheese, ground cumin, salt, and pepper to the skillet. Stir well to combine.
6. Stuff the bell peppers with the quinoa mixture.
7. Place stuffed bell peppers in a baking dish. Cover with aluminum foil.
8. Bake in the preheated oven for 25-30 minutes, or until the peppers are tender.
9. Remove the foil and bake for an additional 5 minutes to melt the cheese.
10. Serve hot.

Nutritional Information (per serving):

- Calories: 280
- Protein: 10g
- Sodium: 180mg
- Potassium: 500mg
- Total Fat: 8g
- Saturated Fat: 3g
- Cholesterol: 10mg
- Carbohydrates: 44g
- Fiber: 7g
- Sugars: 5g

Chicken and Vegetable Stir-Fry

Prep Time: 15 minutes

Cooking Time: 15 minutes

Serving Size: 1 plate

Ingredients:

- 4 oz chicken breast, thinly sliced
- 1 cup mixed vegetables (bell peppers, broccoli, carrots, snap peas)
- 1 clove garlic, minced
- 1 tbsp soy sauce
- 1 tbsp hoisin sauce
- 1/2 tsp sesame oil
- Cooked brown rice for serving

Instructions:

1. Heat sesame oil in a large skillet or wok over medium-high heat.
2. Add minced garlic to the skillet. Cook for 1 minute until fragrant.
3. Add sliced chicken breast to the skillet. Stir-fry for 4-5 minutes until chicken is cooked through.
4. Add mixed vegetables to the skillet. Stir-fry for 4-5 minutes until vegetables are tender-crisp.
5. In a small bowl, mix together soy sauce and hoisin sauce. Pour the sauce mixture over the chicken and vegetables in the skillet.
6. Stir well to combine and coat evenly.
7. Serve the stir-fry hot over cooked brown rice.

Nutritional Information (per serving):

- Calories: 320
- Protein: 28g
- Sodium: 650mg
- Potassium: 620mg
- Total Fat: 7g
- Saturated Fat: 1g
- Cholesterol: 70mg
- Carbohydrates: 38g
- Fiber: 5g
- Sugars: 7g

Lentil and Vegetable Soup

Prep Time: 15 minutes

Cooking Time: 30 minutes

Serving Size: 1 bowl

Ingredients:

- 1/2 cup dried lentils, rinsed
- 4 cups vegetable broth
- 1 carrot, diced
- 1 celery stalk, diced
- 1/2 onion, diced
- 1 clove garlic, minced
- 1 tsp olive oil
- 1/2 tsp dried thyme
- 1/2 tsp dried rosemary
- Salt and pepper to taste
- Chopped fresh parsley for garnish

Instructions:

1. Heat olive oil in a large pot over medium heat.
2. Add diced onion, carrot, and celery to the pot. Cook until softened, about 5 minutes.
3. Add minced garlic, dried thyme, and dried rosemary to the pot. Cook for another minute until fragrant.
4. Add rinsed lentils and vegetable broth to the pot. Bring to a boil.

5. Reduce heat to low, cover, and simmer for 25-30 minutes, or until lentils are tender.

6. Season with salt and pepper to taste.

7. Ladle the soup into bowls and garnish with chopped fresh parsley.

8. Serve hot.

Nutritional Information (per serving):

- Calories: 250

- Protein: 15g

- Sodium: 780mg

- Potassium: 600mg

- Total Fat: 2g

- Saturated Fat: 0g

- Cholesterol: 0mg

- Carbohydrates: 45g

- Fiber: 16g

- Sugars: 6g

Mediterranean Grilled Vegetable Platter

Prep Time: 15 minutes

Cooking Time: 15 minutes

Serving Size: 1 plate

Ingredients:

- 1 small eggplant, sliced

- 1 zucchini, sliced

- 1 yellow squash, sliced

- 1 red bell pepper, sliced
- 1 yellow bell pepper, sliced
- 1 red onion, sliced
- 2 tbsp olive oil
- 2 cloves garlic, minced
- 1 tsp dried oregano
- 1 tsp dried basil
- Salt and pepper to taste
- Lemon wedges for garnish

Instructions:

1. Preheat grill to medium-high heat.
2. In a large bowl, toss sliced eggplant, zucchini, yellow squash, red bell pepper, yellow bell pepper, and red onion with olive oil, minced garlic, dried oregano, dried basil, salt, and pepper.
3. Place the seasoned vegetables on the preheated grill.
4. Grill the vegetables for 4-5 minutes per side, or until they are tender and lightly charred.
5. Remove the grilled vegetables from the grill and arrange them on a serving platter.
6. Garnish with lemon wedges.
7. Serve hot or at room temperature.

Nutritional Information (per serving):

- Calories: 180
- Protein: 4g
- Sodium: 15mg
- Potassium: 700mg

- Total Fat: 14g

- Saturated Fat: 2g

- Cholesterol: 0mg

- Carbohydrates: 15g

- Fiber: 6g

- Sugars: 8g

Turkey and Vegetable Skewers

Prep Time: 20 minutes

Cooking Time: 15 minutes

Serving Size: 1 skewer

Ingredients:

- 8 oz turkey breast, cut into cubes

- zucchini, cut into chunks

- 1 yellow bell pepper, cut into chunks

- 1 red onion, cut into chunks

- 8 cherry tomatoes

- 2 tbsp olive oil

- 2 cloves garlic, minced

- 1 tsp dried thyme

- 1 tsp dried rosemary

- Salt and pepper to taste

Instructions:

1. If using wooden skewers, soak them in water for 30 minutes to prevent burning.

2. In a large bowl, combine turkey breast cubes, zucchini chunks, yellow bell pepper chunks, red onion chunks, cherry tomatoes, olive oil, minced garlic, dried thyme, dried rosemary, salt, and pepper. Toss well to coat.

3. Thread the marinated turkey and vegetables onto skewers, alternating between different ingredients.

4. Preheat grill to medium-high heat.

5. Place the skewers on the preheated grill.

6. Grill the skewers for 10-12 minutes, turning occasionally, until the turkey is cooked through and the vegetables are tender.

7. Remove the skewers from the grill and serve hot.

Nutritional Information (per serving):

- Calories: 220
- Protein: 22g
- Sodium: 55mg
- Potassium: 570mg
- Total Fat: 12g
- Saturated Fat: 2g
- Cholesterol: 55mg
- Carbohydrates: 9g
- Fiber: 3g
- Sugars: 5g

Cauliflower Fried Rice

Prep Time: 15 minutes

Cooking Time: 15 minutes

Serving Size: 1 plate

Ingredients:

- 1 small head cauliflower, grated (or 4 cups cauliflower rice)
- 2 eggs, beaten
- 1 cup mixed vegetables (peas, carrots, corn)
- 2 green onions, thinly sliced
- 2 cloves garlic, minced
- 2 tbsp low-sodium soy sauce
- 1 tbsp sesame oil
- 1 tbsp olive oil
- Salt and pepper to taste

Instructions:

1. Heat olive oil in a large skillet or wok over medium heat.
2. Add minced garlic and sliced green onions to the skillet. Cook for 1 minute until fragrant.
3. Add beaten eggs to the skillet and scramble until cooked through. Remove from the skillet and set aside.
4. In the same skillet, add cauliflower rice and mixed vegetables. Stir-fry for 5-6 minutes until vegetables are tender.
5. Return the scrambled eggs to the skillet with cauliflower rice and mixed vegetables.
6. Add low-sodium soy sauce and sesame oil to the skillet. Stir well to combine.
7. Cook for another 2-3 minutes, stirring constantly, until everything is heated through.

8. Season with salt and pepper to taste.

9. Serve hot.

Nutritional Information (per serving):

- Calories: 200

- Protein: 9g

- Sodium: 430mg

- Potassium: 620mg

- Total Fat: 12g

- Saturated Fat: 2g

- Cholesterol: 110mg

- Carbohydrates: 15g

- Fiber: 6g

- Sugars: 6g

Baked Chicken Parmesan

Prep Time: 15 minutes

Cooking Time: 25 minutes

Serving Size: 1 chicken breast

Ingredients:

- 2 boneless, skinless chicken breasts

- 1/2 cup whole wheat breadcrumbs

- 1/4 cup grated Parmesan cheese

- 1/2 cup marinara sauce

- 1/2 cup shredded mozzarella cheese

- 1 tbsp olive oil

- 1/2 tsp dried oregano

- 1/2 tsp dried basil
- Salt and pepper to taste

Instructions:

2. Preheat oven to 400°F (200°C). Grease a baking dish with olive oil.
3. In a shallow dish, combine whole wheat breadcrumbs, grated Parmesan cheese, dried oregano, dried basil, salt, and pepper.
4. Coat each chicken breast in the breadcrumb mixture, pressing gently to adhere.
5. Place the coated chicken breasts in the greased baking dish.
6. Bake in the preheated oven for 20 minutes.
7. Remove the baking dish from the oven and spoon marinara sauce over each chicken breast.
8. Sprinkle shredded mozzarella cheese on top of each chicken breast.
9. Return the baking dish to the oven and bake for an additional 5 minutes, or until the cheese is melted and bubbly.
10. Serve hot.

Nutritional Information (per serving):

- Calories: 350
- Protein: 40g
- Sodium: 580mg
- Potassium: 510mg
- Total Fat: 13g
- Saturated Fat: 5g

- Cholesterol: 95mg

- Carbohydrates: 20g

- Fiber: 3g

- Sugars: 3g

Spaghetti Squash with Turkey Bolognese Sauce

Prep Time: 15 minutes

Cooking Time: 1 hour

Serving Size: 1 plate

Ingredients:

- 1 medium spaghetti squash

- 8 oz lean ground turkey

- 1 cup marinara sauce

- 1/2 onion, diced

- 1 clove garlic, minced

- 1 tbsp olive oil

- 1/2 tsp dried basil

- 1/2 tsp dried oregano

- Salt and pepper to taste

- Fresh basil leaves for garnish

Instructions:

1. Preheat oven to 375°F (190°C).

2. Cut the spaghetti squash in half lengthwise and scoop out the seeds.

3. Drizzle olive oil over the cut sides of the squash halves and season with salt and pepper.

4. Place the squash halves, cut side down, on a baking sheet lined with parchment paper.

5. Bake in the preheated oven for 45-50 minutes, or until the squash is tender and easily pierced with a fork.

6. While the squash is baking, heat olive oil in a skillet over medium heat.

7. Add diced onion and minced garlic to the skillet. Cook until softened, about 5 minutes.

8. Add ground turkey to the skillet and cook until browned, breaking it into small pieces with a spoon.

9. Stir in marinara sauce, dried basil, dried oregano, salt, and pepper. Simmer for 10-15 minutes.

10. Once the spaghetti squash is cooked, use a fork to scrape the flesh into spaghetti-like strands.

11. Divide the spaghetti squash strands into serving plates and top with turkey bolognese sauce.

12. Garnish with fresh basil leaves.

13. Serve hot.

Nutritional Information (per serving):

- Calories: 320
- Protein: 20g
- Sodium: 530mg
- Potassium: 870mg
- Total Fat: 15g
- Saturated Fat: 3g
- Cholesterol: 50mg

- Carbohydrates: 30g

- Fiber: 6g

- Sugars: 12g

Broccoli and Cheese Stuffed Chicken Breast

Prep Time: 20 minutes

Cooking Time: 25 minutes

Serving Size: 1 stuffed chicken breast

Ingredients:

- 2 boneless, skinless chicken breasts

- 1 cup broccoli florets, steamed

- 1/2 cup shredded cheddar cheese

- 2 tbsp plain Greek yogurt

- 1/4 tsp garlic powder

- 1/4 tsp onion powder

- Salt and pepper to taste

- Olive oil cooking spray

Instructions:

1. Preheat oven to 375°F (190°C). Grease a baking dish with olive oil cooking spray.

2. Butterfly each chicken breast by slicing horizontally through the thickest part, but not all the way through, to create a pocket.

3. In a bowl, mix together steamed broccoli florets, shredded cheddar cheese, plain Greek yogurt, garlic powder, onion powder, salt, and pepper.

4. Stuff each chicken breast with the broccoli and cheese mixture, then secure with toothpicks if needed.

5. Place the stuffed chicken breasts in the greased baking dish.

6. Bake in the preheated oven for 20-25 minutes, or until the chicken is cooked through and no longer pink in the center.

7. Remove the toothpicks before serving.

8. Serve hot

Nutritional Information (per serving):

- Calories: 280
- Protein: 38g
- Sodium: 320mg
- Potassium: 610mg
- Total Fat: 10g
- Saturated Fat: 5g
- Cholesterol: 110mg
- Carbohydrates: 6g
- Fiber: 2g
- Sugars: 2g

SNACKS RECIPES

Avocado and Tomato Bruschetta

Prep Time: 10 minutes

Cooking Time: 5 minutes

Serving Size: 2 slices

Ingredients:

- 2 slices whole grain bread
- 1 ripe avocado, mashed
- 1 medium tomato, diced
- 1 clove garlic, minced
- 1 tablespoon fresh basil, chopped
- 1 tablespoon balsamic vinegar
- Salt and pepper to taste

Instructions:

1. Preheat oven broiler. Place bread slices on a baking sheet and toast under the broiler for 2-3 minutes per side, until golden brown.
2. In a small bowl, mix together mashed avocado, diced tomato, minced garlic, chopped basil, and balsamic vinegar. Season with salt and pepper.
3. Spread the avocado mixture evenly onto the toasted bread slices.
4. Serve immediately.

Nutritional Information (per serving):

- Calories: 158

- Protein: 4g

- Sodium: 195mg

- Potassium: 436mg

- Total Fat: 9g

- Saturated Fat: 1g

- Cholesterol: 0mg

- Carbohydrates: 19g

- Fiber: 7g

- Sugars: 3g

Greek Yogurt and Berry Parfait

Prep Time: 5 minutes

Serving Size: 1 parfait

Ingredients:

- 1/2 cup plain Greek yogurt

- 1/4 cup mixed berries (such as strawberries, blueberries, raspberries)

- 1 tablespoon honey or maple syrup

- 1 tablespoon granola

Instructions:

1. In a glass or bowl, layer half of the Greek yogurt.

2. Add half of the mixed berries on top of the yogurt.

3. Drizzle with half of the honey or maple syrup.

4. Repeat the layers with the remaining yogurt, berries, and sweetener.

5. Sprinkle granola on top just before serving.

Nutritional Information (per serving):

- Calories: 180
- Protein: 14g
- Sodium: 50mg
- Potassium: 230mg
- Total Fat: 4g
- Saturated Fat: 0g
- Cholesterol: 10mg
- Carbohydrates: 26g
- Fiber: 3g
- Sugars: 18g

Turkey and Cheese Roll-Ups

Prep Time: 10 minutes

Serving Size: 2 roll-ups

Ingredients:

- 2 slices turkey breast
- 2 slices low-fat cheese (such as cheddar or Swiss)
- 1/4 avocado, sliced
- 1/2 cucumber, julienned
- 2 large lettuce leaves

Instructions:

1. Lay lettuce leaves flat and place one slice of turkey on each leaf.
2. Top each turkey slice with a slice of cheese, avocado slices, and julienned cucumber.

3. Roll up the lettuce leaves tightly to form a roll-up.

4. Secure with toothpicks if needed.

5. Repeat with the remaining ingredients to make a second roll-up.

6. Serve immediately or refrigerate until ready to eat.

Nutritional Information (per serving):

- Calories: 190

- Protein: 18g

- Sodium: 310mg

- Potassium: 480mg

- Total Fat: 10g

- Saturated Fat: 3g

- Cholesterol: 35mg

- Carbohydrates: 7g

- Fiber: 3g

- Sugars: 2g

Cottage Cheese and Pineapple Bowl

Prep Time: 5 minutes

Serving Size: 1 bowl

Ingredients:

- 1/2 cup low-fat cottage cheese

- 1/2 cup pineapple chunks (fresh or canned in juice)

- tablespoon chopped walnuts or almonds

- 1 teaspoon honey (optional)

Instructions:

1. In a bowl, combine cottage cheese and pineapple chunks.
2. Sprinkle chopped nuts on top.
3. Drizzle with honey if desired.
4. Serve immediately.

Nutritional Information (per serving):

- Calories: 220
- Protein: 20g
- Sodium: 350mg
- Potassium: 330mg
- Total Fat: 6g
- Saturated Fat: 1g
- Cholesterol: 10mg
- Carbohydrates: 22g
- Fiber: 2g
- Sugars: 17g

Veggie Stuffed Bell Peppers

Prep Time: 15 minutes

Cooking Time: 25 minutes

Serving Size: 1 stuffed pepper

Ingredients:

- 1 large bell pepper
- 1/4 cup cooked quinoa or brown rice
- 1/4 cup black beans, drained and rinsed
- 1/4 cup diced tomatoes
- 2 tablespoons diced red onion

- 2 tablespoons chopped cilantro
- 1/2 teaspoon ground cumin
- 1/2 teaspoon chili powder
- Salt and pepper to taste
- 1/4 cup shredded low-fat cheese (optional)

Instructions:

1. Preheat oven to 375°F (190°C).
2. Cut the top off the bell pepper and remove the seeds and membrane.
3. In a bowl, mix together cooked quinoa or brown rice, black beans, diced tomatoes, red onion, cilantro, cumin, chili powder, salt, and pepper.
4. Stuff the mixture into the bell pepper.
5. If using cheese, sprinkle it on top of the stuffed pepper.
6. Place the stuffed pepper on a baking sheet and bake for 25 minutes, or until the pepper is tender.
7. Serve hot.

Nutritional Information (per serving):

- Calories: 180
- Protein: 9g
- Sodium: 270mg
- Potassium: 450mg
- Total Fat: 2g
- Saturated Fat: 0g
- Cholesterol: 0mg
- Carbohydrates: 34g

- Fiber: 8g
- Sugars: 6g

CHAPTER 6

28 DAYS MEAL PLAN

Week 1:

Day 1:

- **Breakfast:** Banana Oat Pancakes
- **Lunch:** Greek Salad with Grilled Chicken
- **Dinner:** Baked Salmon with Roasted Vegetables

Day 2:

- **Breakfast:** Avocado Toast with Poached Eggs
- **Lunch:** Quinoa Salad with Chickpeas and Veggies
- **Dinner:** Spaghetti Aglio e Olio with Garlic Bread

Day 3:

- **Breakfast**: Berry Smoothie Bowl
- **Lunch:** Turkey and Veggie Wrap with Hummus
- **Dinner:** Veggie Stir-Fry with Tofu and Brown Rice

Day 4:

- **Breakfast:** Veggie Omelette with Whole Grain Toast
- **Lunch:** Lentil Soup with Whole Grain Bread
- **Dinner**: Grilled Shrimp Tacos with Mango Salsa

Day 5:

- Breakfast: Yogurt Parfait with Granola and Fresh Fruit
- **Lunch:** Caprese Sandwich with Tomato Soup
- **Dinner:** Stuffed Bell Peppers with Quinoa and Black Beans

Day 6:

- **Breakfast:** Spinach and Feta Frittata

- **Lunch:** Chicken Caesar Salad

- **Dinner:** Teriyaki Chicken with Steamed Broccoli and Rice

Day 7:

- **Breakfast:** Overnight Chia Seed Pudding with Berries

- **Lunch:** Mediterranean Veggie Bowl with Hummus

- **Dinner:** Vegetable Lasagna with Garlic Bread

Week 2:

Day 8:

- **Breakfast:** Blueberry Banana Smoothie

- **Lunch:** Tuna Salad Sandwich with Whole Grain Crackers

- **Dinner:** Baked Chicken Parmesan with Mixed Greens Salad

Day 9:

- **Breakfast:** Breakfast Burrito with Salsa

- **Lunch:** Quinoa Stuffed Bell Peppers

- **Dinner:** Shrimp Scampi with Whole Wheat Pasta

Day 10:

- **Breakfast: Greek Yogurt with Honey and Nuts**

- **Lunch: Black Bean and Corn Quesadillas**

- **Dinner: Thai Basil Beef Stir-Fry with Jasmine Rice**

Day 11:

- **Breakfast:** Whole Wheat Waffles with Fresh Fruit

- **Lunch:** Veggie and Hummus Wrap

- **Dinner:** Baked Cod with Lemon Herb Butter and Roasted Potatoes

Day 12:

- **Breakfast:** Veggie Breakfast Hash with Poached Eggs
- **Lunch:** Asian Noodle Salad with Peanut Dressing
- **Dinner:** Chicken Fajitas with Guacamole and Corn Tortillas

Day 13:

- **Breakfast:** Oatmeal with Almond Butter and Banana Slices
- **Lunch:** Chickpea Salad with Cucumber and Feta
- **Dinner:** Eggplant Parmesan with Spaghetti Squash

Day 14:

- **Breakfast**: Scrambled Tofu with Spinach and Tomatoes
- **Lunch:** Quinoa and Black Bean Salad
- **Dinner:** Beef and Broccoli Stir-Fry with Brown Rice

Week 3:

Day 15:

- **Breakfast:** Mixed Berry Smoothie with Protein Powder
- **Lunch:** Mediterranean Couscous Salad
- **Dinner:** Baked Lemon Herb Chicken with Roasted Vegetables

Day 16:

- **Breakfast**: Breakfast Burrito Bowl with Avocado
- **Lunch:** Lentil and Vegetable Soup with Whole Grain Bread
- **Dinner:** Grilled Steak with Chimichurri Sauce and Sweet Potato Fries

Day 17:

- **Breakfast:** Chia Seed Pudding with Mango and Coconut
- **Lunch:** Spinach and Strawberry Salad with Balsamic Vinaigrette
- **Dinner:** Vegetable Curry with Basmati Rice

Day 18:

- **Breakfast:** Peanut Butter Banana Toast
- **Lunch:** Quinoa and Vegetable Stir-Fry
- **Dinner:** Salmon with Dill Sauce and Steamed Asparagus

Day 19:

- **Breakfast:** Whole Grain Pancakes with Maple Syrup and Berries
- **Lunch:** Caprese Pasta Salad
- **Dinner:** Turkey Meatballs with Marinara Sauce and Zucchini Noodles

Day 20:

- **Breakfast:** Avocado and Egg Breakfast Sandwich
- **Lunch:** Black Bean Burrito Bowl with Salsa and Guacamole
- **Dinner:** Teriyaki Tofu with Stir-Fried Vegetables and Brown Rice

Day 21:

- **Breakfast:** Greek Yogurt Parfait with Granola and Honey
- Lunch: **Chickpea and Avocado Salad**
- **Dinner:** Vegetable Enchiladas with Mexican Rice

Week 4:

Day 22:

- **Breakfast:** Berry and Spinach Smoothie
- **Lunch:** Quinoa and Black Bean Wrap with Avocado
- **Dinner:** Grilled Chicken Caesar Salad

Day 23:

- **Breakfast:** Banana Nut Overnight Oats
- **Lunch:** Mediterranean Veggie Pizza
- **Dinner:** Baked Cod with Tomato and Olive Relish and Quinoa Pilaf

Day 24:

- **Breakfast:** Veggie Breakfast Burrito with Salsa
- **Lunch:** Thai Peanut Noodle Salad
- **Dinner:** Beef and Vegetable Kabobs with Tzatziki Sauce and Couscous

Day 25:

- **Breakfast:** Spinach and Mushroom Frittata
- **Lunch**: Lentil and Vegetable Curry with Naan Bread
- **Dinner:** Honey Mustard Glazed Salmon with Roasted Brussels Sprouts

Day 26:

- **Breakfast:** Whole Wheat French Toast with Berries
- **Lunch:** Greek Salad with Grilled Shrimp
- **Dinner: Vegetable** Stir-Fry with Tofu and Quinoa

Day 27:

- **Breakfast:** Yogurt and Fruit Smoothie Bowl

- **Lunch:** Caprese Sandwich with Minestrone Soup
- **Dinner:** Spaghetti Squash with Marinara Sauce and Turkey Meatballs

Day 28:

- **Breakfast:** Oatmeal with Almond Butter and Sliced Banana
- **Lunch:** Black Bean and Corn Quesadillas with Guacamole
- **Dinner:** Chicken Stir-Fry with Bell Peppers and Brown Rice

CONCLUSION

In conclusion, the "Carb Cycling Cookbook for Seniors" offers a tailored approach to nutrition that aligns with the unique needs of older adults. By combining the principles of carb cycling with recipes specifically designed for seniors, this cookbook provides a comprehensive resource for maintaining health and vitality in later years.

The diverse array of recipes ensures that seniors can enjoy a variety of delicious meals while effectively managing their carbohydrate intake. This approach not only supports energy levels and overall well-being but also addresses potential concerns such as blood sugar management and weight control.

Moreover, the emphasis on nutrient-dense ingredients, balanced meals, and appropriate portion sizes reflects a holistic approach to senior nutrition. By incorporating whole grains, lean proteins, healthy fats, and plenty of fruits and vegetables, the cookbook promotes optimal health and supports healthy aging.

Overall, the "Carb Cycling Cookbook for Seniors" serves as a valuable tool for older adults looking to enhance their nutrition, maintain an active lifestyle, and thrive in their golden years. With its practical guidance and delicious recipes, it empowers seniors to take control of their health and enjoy a fulfilling culinary experience.

In summary, the "Carb Cycling Cookbook for Seniors" provides a tailored nutritional approach for older adults, offering a diverse range of recipes specifically designed to meet their needs. By emphasizing balanced meals, appropriate portion sizes, and nutrient-dense ingredients, this cookbook promotes optimal health and supports healthy aging. With its practical guidance and delicious recipes, it serves as a valuable resource for seniors looking to enhance their nutrition, maintain an active lifestyle, and enjoy flavorful meals tailored to their dietary requirements.s